Today's date: _____

Name: ___Abigail Calumpit_____

Course name, working project, or thesis title or theme: _____

_____

If this guide is found, contact me at: ___(718) 755 - 6028_____

_____abigail.calumpit@gmail.com_____

_____

_____

_____

DOING DEVELOPMENTAL RESEARCH

DOING DEVELOPMENTAL RESEARCH

A Practical Guide

Tricia Striano

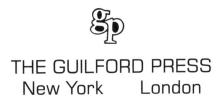

THE GUILFORD PRESS
New York   London

Library of Congress Cataloging-in-Publication Data

Names: Striano, Tricia, author.
Title: Doing developmental research : a practical guide / by Tricia Striano.
Description: New York : The Guilford Press, [2016] | Includes bibliographical
    references and index.
Identifiers: LCCN 2015048258| ISBN 9781462524426 (paperback) | ISBN
    9781462524433 (hardcover)
Subjects: LCSH: Developmental psychology—Research—Methodology. | Child
    development—Research—Methodology. | Report writing. | BISAC: SOCIAL
    SCIENCE / Research. | MEDICAL / Nursing / Research & Theory. | PSYCHOLOGY
    / Developmental / General. | EDUCATION / Research.
Classification: LCC BF713 .S766 2016 | DDC 150.72/1—dc23
LC record available at http://lccn.loc.gov/2015048258

Preface

Why a guide on how to get research done?

This guide is designed to assist undergraduate and graduate students in achieving their research goals and completing their research projects, theses, and dissertations more effectively by streamlining the process of research.

In designing this book, I selected materials from laboratories around the globe and from researchers at different stages of their careers. I focus on many aspects of research not typically considered in standard research methods books such as how to recruit participants for infant or child development studies and how to publish your results effectively by better understanding the submission and review process for journals. The recruitment of study participants, data management methods, and institutional review board issues, as well as the best paradigms and coding schemes to use, are some common issues that arise when you conduct research.

Almost everything in this guide I learned from or developed with those who trained, guided, and supported or inspired me during my research career. I have been blessed with wonderful mentors, colleagues, students, supportive parents, and a couple of great secretaries who cared for and taught me along the way. I hope to have given them proper credit throughout this guide and, most importantly, shared much of what they taught me along the way. Special thanks to many of my mentors and close collaborators: Danuta Bukatko, Philippe Rochat, Angela Friederici, Patricia Brennan, Roseanne Flores, Sheila Chase, Virginia Valian, Sabine Pauen, Heidi Keller, Daniel Stahl, Vincent Reid, Stefanie Hoehl, Eugenio Parise, Mariah Schug, Allison Cleveland, Roberta Fadda, and my former secretaries Bettina Wollesky and Filu Howey. I am grateful to the Max Planck Society for supporting my early research career, providing me the opportunity for a steep learning curve at the Max Planck Institute for Evolutionary Anthropology and the Max Planck Institute for Human Cognitive and Brain Sciences. I am grateful to the Alexander von Humboldt Foundation for supporting several grants and awards, including the Sofja Kovalevskaja Award, which allowed me to develop innovative and highly international research teams. Thank you for providing the infrastructure and resources for *Doing Developmental Research*! I am thankful to many students and colleagues at Hunter College, The City University of New York, for inspiring this book. The development of the manuscript was helped by the guidance of Guilford's anonymous reviewers, whose names were revealed to me upon completion of the final version. My thanks to the following people for their insights and thoughtful comments: Melissa Y. Delgado, School of Family and Consumer Sciences, Texas State University; Catherine A. Forestall, Department of Psychology, College of William and Mary; and Yvette R. Harris, Center for School-Based Mental Health Programs, Miami University.

The strategies and methods in this book are often used in my own laboratory. I have had the opportunity to pursue research in diverse environments, and from these very broad experiences I learned that research can be done in a variety of contexts. When planning your research, you have to determine your unique resources, plan ahead, and be strategic and creative to get it done most efficiently and effectively.

As your research career progresses, so will your skills and strategies. Many tips were developed in the context of a full teaching load that included undergraduate courses on research methods, cognitive development, and developmental methods, and especially from working with hundreds of undergraduate and graduate students over the past several years.

A guide to facilitate research

This is not a research methods book but rather a practical guide that focuses on the process of getting research done effectively. I assume that, by the time you pick up this book, you have taken a course in basic research methodology and statistics (and have reviewed these subjects recently if you are planning to generate statistics in your study). We can become forgetful of details—especially if we do not regularly apply our knowledge and skills. If you have not reviewed statistics recently, now is the time to do so. If you are being interviewed to work in a social sciences research laboratory (or any laboratory), you should not be asking, "Will I need to know statistics?" *Of course* you will need to have a basic understanding of statistics. You cannot understand any research paper if you do not have a basic background in statistics. You should want to have some knowledge of the subject even if you do not select a career in research. After all, it is useful in investing in the stock market, deciding whether to buy or rent a home, or forecasting which team will win the World Cup. By becoming actively involved in a research laboratory, you will gain the opportunity to practice and apply statistics much more rigorously.

How to use this guide

If you are new to research laboratories or just starting a thesis or project, you might wish to read this entire guide first and then return to individual sections as needed. Efficient research often involves working on several aspects of your research projects simultaneously.

For example, while writing up your thesis proposal, you might already be researching schools, parks, and events at which you could recruit children for your studies in the developmental sciences. Even if your research study and recruitment plans have not yet been approved by the institutional review board of your university, you may already be thinking about how to locate your research participants. For example, you can begin developing lists of schools and day care centers, start purchasing toys and stimuli that you will use in your study, and further plan, prepare, and strategize. You should get familiar with the locality that you are in and develop a basic plan and strategy for recruiting participants for your study. It is done differently, after all, in the heart of a major city versus in a rural location, so get a feel for your specific location. This is not accomplished by sitting behind a computer or searching the Internet, but rather by getting out into the community. Notice *where* your target participants tend to congregate. From supermarkets to gyms, churches, parks, and the beach, begin to get a feel for the resources around you. Even while your mentor is first reading your thesis proposal, you can begin designing basic flyers to promote your research study, planning recruitment strategies, or compiling materials such as toys that you will likely need to run your research study. You might also begin to familiarize yourself with specialized equipment that you may be using and run a "mock" study. In the process, you may discover that you do not know the password for a particular computer or perhaps that a software license has expired. Research is a process of problem solving and problem prevention. Like development, research is not always a linear step-by-step process. In the process of conducting research, you should always strive to "keep it simple." This guide will assist you in asking your research questions in a direct and concise way so that you can answer them effectively and then publish your findings.

If you are a more advanced student, you can use this guide to develop time management strategies for organizing and conducting several studies at once. I have included tips for writing up your research papers and dealing with comments from reviewers. Sections on ethics and authorship may also be helpful as your research network expands or as you seek solutions to common problems that arise in the process of research. Use this guide to plan your research strategies and to predict and prevent problems *before* they occur. I have included numerous blank spaces for your input on purpose. As a researcher, you sometimes need to go back to the drawing boards to make changes in your ideas and protocols. It is wise to keep your notes in one secure location and to build upon your prior discussions and ideas.

At this point, you should purchase a notebook for your research and research-related activities. Carry this notebook with you at all times, and jot your research ideas in it. Date the cover of the notebook and all your entries. Use it only for your research. Be sure to always bring your notebook/log when you have meetings about research. Although it is now common to use a phone or digital device to take notes, there are several advantages to also writing in a dedicated log or notebook. An old-fashioned paper notebook is less likely to be stolen, lost, or broken. Another advantage is that the notebook can be shared by others on your team with ease. For example, when I meet with the students in my laboratory, I often have recommendations. Sometimes we want to draw diagrams or make notes that can be referred to and relocated easily in the future. A paper notebook allows for such flexibility. An old-fashioned paper notebook also does not lead to distractions (whether beeps, apps, or rings) that might divert us away from the more relevant aspects of research. Now that you have your notebook, let's begin discussing the first steps in getting involved in research. One of your first tasks is to assess what research topics most excite you.

Contents

Purchasers of this book can download and print
enlarged versions of select forms
at *www.guilford.com/striano-forms* for personal use.

CHAPTER 1

Selecting a Laboratory

No matter WHAT research you wish to explore, almost immediately you will want to select a laboratory. Because I supervise a laboratory in the developmental sciences, many examples cited in this volume are derived from this field. Whatever your exact academic discipline, however, the same principles and strategies should apply. You want to begin to think like a researcher as you start choosing what subject you want to explore.

So, why might I want to study infant and child development in a laboratory setting?

(The answer should not be "Because I think children are cute" or "I enjoy babysitting.") One key reason to work in a laboratory is to gain relevant experience in research so that you can effectively answer questions about development or your particular research question. During early human development, some of the most rapid changes occur. This is one reason that researchers choose to study the mechanisms of developmental change in human infants and children. When a baby is born, he or she cannot speak, crawl, or use words to communicate his or her thoughts and desires. Several months later the baby can walk and point to show you something, and he or she will eventually say, "Now, I want juice!" How did this transformation occur? What experiences were necessary? Were there critical points in the development? What roles did genetic and biological factors play? Of course, there are special demands and crucial things to know when working with infants and children.

One of the main reasons to study development is because you are interested in the mechanisms of change. Change occurs across contexts, and thus development is relevant whether you want to become a nurse, an economist, a psychiatrist, or a teacher. How did we get from point A to C or Z, and how can we learn from time and changes to solve problems more effectively? Perhaps you are interested in the brain changes that occur as people age. Perhaps you want to know how the latest behavioral therapy for autism influences social behavior as a function of age. Maybe you want to know how social media influences mood or learning. It is difficult to think of a research question that does not involve development to some degree. Although this guide focuses on some issues particular to studying infants and children, I hope that you might learn from the tips regardless of your exact research discipline and field.

> One of the most amazing qualities of living organisms is their incredible capacity for change. Change occurs throughout the lifespan, but is especially dramatic in the first few years of life as children learn to cope with the physical and social environment in an adaptive way. I study development because I am interested in processes of change and adaptation.
> —Kari Kretch, PhD candidate, Department of Psychology, New York University

Why development?

> If you study child development, you can choose among all topics that are relevant for psychology in general. Just add the dimensions of time, and focus on relevant changes. It is the changes that I am interested in! Most changes in human development occur during infancy—that's one important reason why I became an infant researcher.
> I have always been fascinated by the question of how human thinking develops in the first place—when we still don't have any "language of thought." If you want to explore preverbal thinking, you need to start very early—during the first year of life.
> Another reason to study development is that it is fun! Intellectually, it provides a great challenge to study infants' mental processes. Designing experiments to find out more about it often requires me to design new toys and displays, and this combination

of creating something with your hands as well as with your mind is
highly rewarding!
        —Professor Dr. Sabina Pauen, Professor of Psychology, Heidelberg University

What will I gain with laboratory experience?

There are several advantages to becoming involved in a research laboratory. You will gain important hands-on experience and learn about the
research process along the way. There are so many aspects of research
that are often not revealed in textbooks or classes. You will learn to
work on a team, be introduced to new research, and have the opportunity to discuss your ideas with other researchers. You may discover
that you truly enjoy research, and this knowledge could help you make
decisions about your potential career or graduate studies. Working in
a laboratory also opens up many networking opportunities, especially
if it has ongoing partnerships and collaborations in other parts of the
world. Thus, not only will you likely have the opportunity to develop
new skills there but also to network and collaborate with new people
and research teams. As a research student in a laboratory, you gain
opportunities to present your research at university events and conferences and ultimately even to publish your research findings in journals. You also learn a great deal just by observing and helping your
teammates and more senior researchers. Whether you are attending a
practice conference talk of a lab mate or helping to greet participants as
they enter the laboratory, you are learning about the process of research
along the way. In addition, joining a laboratory may give you direct and
immediate access to information on conferences, graduate schools, and
even possible funding opportunities. The partnerships that you develop
may result in fruitful career-long collaborations and friendships.

By participating in a research laboratory, you gain experience working with senior faculty and more experienced researchers. This allows
others to get to know you on a more personal level. This is often helpful
as you seek to develop important references you will need for graduate
school or employment. Graduate schools typically seek out highly recommended, hardworking, and passionate students with direct research
experience. Even if you are not considering graduate school in the social
sciences, almost all careers involve research to some degree. Whether
you are interested in medicine, law, finance, starting up your own business, or even deciding which brand of television to purchase (or whom

to marry), research skills can't hurt! In sum, becoming involved in a research laboratory can give you many of the skills that you will need in life and may also help pave the way as you make various career and education decisions.

What are some of the qualities I will need to get research done?

In part, the answer to this question depends on your chosen research field. To conduct developmental research effectively, you often need to network and market yourself constantly. You need to understand the importance of the research you are conducting and to communicate its relevance to parents and the community in which you are working. You will need a great deal of patience, time, and (often) creativity. Whether you are an undergraduate student just getting started with research or a more advanced researcher, this guide should help you get started. Much like a baby or child, you should have a completely open mind as you begin conducting research. It is easy to think that you should be certain about your future career—especially during your undergraduate years. You may look at your professors, colleagues, and mentors and read their journal articles and think, "This researcher must have always been sure he or she wanted to study child development!" My students are always a bit surprised to learn that this is not always the case. As an undergraduate student, I was never interested in studying infants or early human development. I thought I wanted to be a pathologist or perhaps a surgeon—until I nearly fainted in a hospital (as a visitor)! I was interested in pathology mainly because I enjoyed being a detective. To be a capable scientist and researcher you need to be a good detective. The more complex the case and the more mysterious the question, the more exciting it is to discover answers. If you are a pathologist, you cannot ask your patients what they are thinking or feeling, but yet you have to figure out how they got from A to Z (death). Regardless of the given field, development often gives the detective clues and answers.

Am I prepared to do research?

Only you know the answer to this question. Keep an open mind, because you never know what you will discover as you pursue research.

You will need to have an open mind as you approach your research and even as you interact with your data. Sometimes your theories and ideas prove incorrect. This is often one of the most exciting parts of research. To be an effective researcher you need to be flexible, open to surprises and possibilities. Think like a baby and child by remaining persistent, curious, and open-minded.

Are there certain qualities I will need to be a good researcher?

The answer to this question largely depends on the field of research you have chosen, but, whatever your choice, you need to be passionate. If you want to study early infant and child development, you need to be a good detective and a sensitive person. Like a baby lacking speech, you often may need to have better nonverbal than verbal skills. The same is probably true if you study animals. You need to tune into their needs, feelings, and desires without relying on spoken language. In the field of infant development, in addition to the needs of parents and children, you have to be sensitive to and open to the needs and goals of educators, doctors, nurses, and day care providers. This is especially true if you are working with children with special needs and communicative impairments. I've tested thousands of babies over the years and worked with hundreds of students and researchers at all levels. From this experience I learned that you need to be able to put yourself in the shoes of a parent, an infant, and a child. **Whatever your chosen field, put yourself in the shoes (or paws, cage, fish tank, etc.) of your subject.**

When should I begin to look for a mentor or research supervisor?

Begin searching for a mentor early on, as faculty members typically receive dozens of such requests each semester. Like many researchers, I generally begin getting together my research team for the fall semester in February and March. Keep in mind that semesters begin at different times around the world. You may not receive the same reply from a scholar in the United States versus Italy, if you write in August. Be aware of the cultural contexts and semester schedules for various universities.

Try to "think outside of the box" if a mentor is not available at your university. What connections do you have that may help you to find a mentor? Tell your friends, family members, and professors what you are seeking. You might even consider using social media for your search. Once I met a gentleman from Missouri at a reception in New York City, and his daughter living in Chicago later became a research assistant in my laboratory for the summer. This never would have happened had her father not known that she was seeking a research internship experience. Network broadly and persistently, and always be professional. Attending talks, events, and conferences can also be a great method of finding a potential mentor. When you attend a conference or research event, you should consider reaching out to a potential mentor in advance to see if you could meet informally for coffee and to discuss your interests and possible opportunities. Also, even look outside of your university if possible. Often you may find relevant events taking place at local museums, schools, meet-up groups, hospitals, and libraries.

How can I find a research advisor?

Most often, you can find a research advisor at your university. However, in many cases that may not be possible. For instance, you may be at a small college, or perhaps your research interests do not match the interests of potential advisors. In this case, you may want to begin by asking your professors whom they would recommend to advise you. Often your professors have a broad network of colleagues and may be able to suggest some possibilities. If this approach proves unsuccessful, however, you might also wish to contact outside researchers directly. If you do so, be specific about why you are contacting them, and do some serious vetting beforehand. If you are interested in working with someone special, show him or her that you have read their own research. Rather than merely stating that you enjoy working with children, show that you know the relevant research and explain why you wish to be further involved in it. Always be sure to use the direct address. When I receive an email reading "Dear Professor: I am a sophomore and interested in getting research experience with children. Can you let me know if you have volunteer openings in your lab?," typically I delete it. You may wish to show a mentor or professor or professional your cover letter if you are unsure what to write. Take time to thank others for their time and be professional, and they will be happy to guide you. When undertaking a search for a research advisor, you might also consider joining professional social networking sites such as LinkedIn or Research Gate and attending local research talks and events.

As with any relationship, the key to finding a good mentor is achieving a good fit. In an ideal relationship, you typically share common interests, goals, beliefs, and a like spirit. A mentor–student relationship shares many of the same characteristics. Just as you may not feel like arguing with a partner about politics or religion, you likely will not wish to constantly argue with your mentor about interpretations or the meaning of the data that you collect. Some researchers have very strong views and theories about their research findings. Just as it is difficult to change one's political or religious views, it can be difficult to change a researcher's position on early development. This is not to say that you should seek out only like-minded mentors, but keep in mind that the mentor–student relationship is just like any other relationship. Your openness and ability to communicate as well as the quality of your relationship will likely influence your productivity, happiness, and future. Ideally, your supervisor benefits from having you in his or her lab, and you benefit from your supervisor's presence and oversight. Common interests, common goals, and a personality that fits are just some of the factors you should consider in seeking out a mentor. You may also find that you just do not "click" with your mentor for one reason or another. Think about the reasons why, and try to develop a strategy or plan for improving the relationship and communication (ideally one that involves face-to-face interaction as opposed to email exchanges) if possible. If that does not work, consider discussing the idea of a different mentor or a comentor who might be a better fit. Honesty is always a great policy.

May I work in your laboratory?

Passion, curiosity, and drive are key to research success. Before you leap into a research project, you should want to understand what you are getting yourself into. Before you begin working in a laboratory, you want to be sure that you are generally familiar with the research that is taking place there. One great way to do that is to read several papers or peruse the website of the laboratory that you are interested in working in. If the lab you are considering does not have publications available, you might try asking for recommended readings from the laboratory. Usually research laboratories sponsor a website in which they list relevant papers and research of theirs that can be downloaded. You might also try using such databases as PsycINFO or Google Scholar to find references. If you are not familiar with how to use various databases for selecting research papers, consider consulting with your university librarian. Libraries often offer complimentary lessons in research basics. The internet is also an excellent resource. For instance, the American Psychological Association (APA) offers a series of tutorials on APA databases that you may find helpful as you search for relevant references. Remember that each research article can take anywhere from 1 to 5 hours to process thoroughly.

Read and try to understand all sections of the relevant papers. Method and results sections help you to understand the research paper and also give you essential background to help you write up your own method and results section when you are preparing your own papers for publication.

If you are having to choose among several laboratories, be sure to read several papers from each laboratory. By the end of this exercise, you will have a better idea of the laboratory that may be the best fit for you. The exercises in this book may also help you. You may have the opportunity to serve a rotation in a laboratory prior to selecting the best fit. This will depend on the particular laboratory and/or your university and research setting. It is also important to remember that infant and child development research is highly interdisciplinary. Whether you are a music major, a computer scientist, or an art major, there is probably a need for you in a laboratory. As a leader of a developmental laboratory, I enjoy working with students from fields as diverse as computer science, music, art, and biology/neurosciences. Think outside of the box as you explore the possibilities.

I can't wait to get started in research! What's my next step?

Once you have selected a possible mentor by using the methods just described, the time has now come to make contact. You should prepare yourself in advance to contact the director of the laboratory you are interested in working in via phone or email. Be sure to be positive and clear about your goals. Set yourself apart from the rest of the competition by being professional and demonstrating that you did your homework. You should examine closely any laboratory application guidelines provided, and follow these precisely. Often these are available on the laboratory's website. I often direct interested students to a graduate student for a preliminary meeting about my laboratory. This can help students who might feel too intimidated by having a preliminary meeting with a faculty advisor. Current lab members are often great judges of character, professionalism, and passion. At the meeting, be sure to act professionally, that is, show up on time, address everyone directly, and wear attire that is professionally correct. It is common to send quick and easy text messages or replies. Show how interested you are by taking the time to send a proper reply or email after your meeting.

 Don't Write:

Dear Dr. Smith,

I am a psychology major aspiring to become an elementary school psychologist. Considering the critical role that early development plays in all aspects of life, I was interested in participating as a research assistant in your infancy research lab. Unfortunately, I read that a 6-month commitment is required. I am getting married in August and going on a 4-week honeymoon, so a commitment of that length would not be possible. Also in late October I am having surgery on my knee, so I will be out of commission for 3 weeks. However, I would appreciate meeting with you to discuss how I can begin to work with you!

Thank you for your consideration.

[Name]

Do Write:

Dear Dr. Smith,

I am a Psychology Major at College X and will be a junior beginning next semester. I have reviewed all of the guidelines that I found at your website, *xxxxx.com*, and believe that your laboratory may be an ideal fit. I also hope to do an honors thesis in my senior year.

I am very interested in early infant learning and have recently read several of your research papers, including "Taking a Closer Look at Social and

Cognitive Skills: A Weekly Longitudinal Assessment between 7 and 10 Months of Age" and "Joint Attention and Object Learning in 5- and 7-Month Old Infants," that I found on your website. I am especially interested in your research showing that babies learn from eye gaze cues as early as 3 months of age.

Might you be available in the next weeks to discuss the possibility of my joining your laboratory? If so, could you let me know your available times? Monday 3–6, Tuesday 9–2, and Wednesday 9–12 are generally best for me. I look forward to hearing back from you.

Sincerely,

[Full name]

Use your academic email address, and indicate which school you attend. Professors and senior researchers often receive several requests from students who write from Gmail, Hotmail, and Yahoo. Researchers receive requests from students from numerous universities and sometimes are not sure whether the student writing attends the university where the researchers are employed. Always try to write from the same email address. You do not want to miss a lab meeting or interview on Monday because someone wrote to your private email address and you only check that account on Wednesday. If you want to make a good first impression, consider using a clear subject heading and a professional email address. Always check your spelling, and use the salutation most common in that environment. For example, if you are writing to a professor in Germany, you might write, "Dear Professor Dr. [last name]"— whereas in the United States you would write, "Dear Professor [last name]." However, whenever you are in doubt about a salutation, opting for the more formal one is advisable.

I have been selected for an interview—now what?

Remember to take your notes and notebook with you on the day of your interview and to ask about researchers' expectations of their assistants in the laboratory. How do you best prepare for your interview? Get to know your schedule ahead of time, and bring a copy of your time availabilities for the next 6–12 months (even listing your weekend availability if possible). I generally expect a minimum commitment of

12 months for my infant and child development laboratory; however, the specifics will depend on the laboratory that you apply for. Child development research often involves a special commitment, because working with and recruiting children is usually very time-consuming. Recruiting babies as well as testing and writing up the subsequent research consumes lots of time. It can be difficult to accomplish much in a laboratory in less than a year or two. No matter what your field, you will want to check with the laboratory you have selected about how it is structured and its required time commitments.

If you do not know your schedule yet or it is "up in the air," then you are probably not ready to begin doing research and to commit to a lab. Put yourself in your professor's or mentor's place. Your mentor wants to solve problems and get research done. That is most likely why he or she selected a career in research. He or she does not want to hear: "I'm being interviewed for a job next week and will know my schedule in 3 weeks. In addition, I have to check about my internship at the hospital and with the other labs that I'm working in."

You will want to demonstrate to any lab that truly interests you that work is your first priority. You have probably heard the saying "Actions speak louder than words." Working in a laboratory is often a full-time undertaking. Professors and researchers are most impressed when students show that they understand the need for genuine commitment, as opposed to explaining that they are working in two, three, or four laboratories or that they hold other internships. The latter response typically shows that a student needs more time to figure out his or her future before committing to anything new. Of course, this depends on the particular laboratory in question. Still you must be certain you have adequate time available in order to make a firm work commitment. To get its research done, it is important that your interests not suddenly change 3–6 months into the lab's long-term research project.

Child development research often demands a bit more planning than research with adults. This is because you will often be constrained by babies' schedules (e.g., when they are awake, when they are not hungry), working parents' ability to bring their children to the laboratory, or children's attending class (if you are testing in schools and educational settings). Many child development laboratories even conduct studies on the weekends and early evenings for this reason. As you prepare for your interview or informational meeting, you should consider what specific questions you have about the laboratory.

Possible Questions for Your Interview

"Who would most directly supervise me [e.g., my professor, a visiting scholar, a postdoc, or an MA student]?"

"Do you test children on the weekends?"

"How do you recruit participants for your studies?"

"Will I get to select my own project, or would you place me on a preexisting project?"

"What readings would you recommend?"

"What are your expectations for an honors student, PhD student, etc.?"

"Does your lab run on the weekends or during the summer?"

When do I need to be available?

You should bring your personal time schedule to your interview so you are not lost when asked, "What days and times are you available?" You will likely want to schedule time commitments in blocks of about 3 hours, as it is usually difficult to accomplish your goals in 1- to 2-hour slots. Check with your prospective supervisor to get more details about how the lab functions.

I was selected for an internship at a highly competitive child development lab for next semester. Is this the right lab for me?

You will likely need some experience to determine which type of lab works best for you. You will need to consider whether your expectations fit with those of the lab. You will want to consider if you are passionate about the type of research being conducted and comfortable with the working dynamics of the laboratory. Do you prefer a larger laboratory with 10–15 projects under way or perhaps a smaller laboratory? From funding to lab location, there are many factors to consider. I always ask potential research assistants and interns to take 2–5 days before deciding if mine is the right laboratory for them. There are major differences when working with children and families, versus adults and animals. One main challenge is that recruiting participants for research takes a very long time and a great deal of marketing and public relations skills. You cannot just go to the university and enlist college students or go into the lab and test a mouse, squirrel, or pigeon. During the early years of starting up a laboratory, on average it takes 1–3 hours to recruit a child for a study and to get him or her into the laboratory. As a lab worker, you will need time, motivation, and passion. Unless you are working with precollected data, you will often need to set aside sizable blocks of time during the day. I have many students who want to be child development researchers but are also working full-time jobs and also taking three to five classes each semester. Know what you are getting yourself into before you commit to research in a laboratory.

It depends on the particular laboratory that you are working in, but I recommend having available a minimum of 20 hours a week for volunteers, those in independent study, and honors students (and more than double that for graduate students and postdoctoral students). This level of commitment allows for about 6 hours of reading research and writing per week; about 4 hours of lab work to test babies or children (which would achieve about two to five data points, given that some parents may have to cancel or babies may become fussy in a study); about 3 hours to set up for studies, obtain materials, and remain organized; 3 hours to recruit to achieve the data points above; 2 hours to meet with the mentor and present at lab meetings, practice for presentations, network, attend relevant talks or events, or submit abstracts for a conference; and about 2 hours to code and analyze the data you collect and to keep your data records organized. Of course, you would need to check the lab guidelines and particular expectations of your mentor, but the foregoing are my own general guidelines.

 When you are ready to commit, let your professor or the person you met in the laboratory know your decision. Otherwise, send them a thank you note for their time. Here is an example of an acceptance note that I received recently that may give you some useful ideas.

Dear Dr. Striano,

I am emailing because I cannot wait to start working with your laboratory. I am going to contact the research doctoral student I am working with to tell her that your laboratory is a better fit for me. I took your advice on focusing on research with your laboratory because it will give me focus, discipline, and structure.

I am completely open with my time; if at all possible, Mon.–Thurs. work best for me. Months back I booked two trips: one in the last week of June: Thurs., June 27–Mon., July 1st. The 2nd is Mon., Sept. 2nd–Sun., Sept. 8th. These are the only time constraints I foresee, and will make sure to work around these. I hope this will not affect my doing research with you.

You asked me what I wanted to focus on, and I would love to study how infants and children may learn from media. I look forward to hearing back from you.

Thank you,

[Name]

Note: I appreciated how this student informed me about her upcoming trip and also let me know about her schedule. In this way, we were better able to begin planning months ahead.

I never heard back from the lab I am interested in working in. What should I do?

If you never received any acknowledgment from the lab that you were interested in working in, you might try resending your request. However, do not take it personally if you do not subsequently hear back from them. There may be several reasons for the omission. Perhaps your mother (if she's like mine) once told you, "The squeaky wheel gets the grease." Sometimes you will need to be persistent. However, at other times a lack of response may indicate that a potential mentor just does not have time for you. Ideally you should find a mentor and laboratory that have time to dedicate to you (and vice versa). If your request is declined by a laboratory, ask for feedback and inquire whether you may check back with them at a later date. You might also try to obtain feedback from the current members of the lab. Do not get discouraged but rather learn from the experience and try to find a different laboratory. You might also consider asking your professors if they are accepting applicants (or if they know who is) at the beginning of the semester.

The tips in this chapter should help you to select the right laboratory for you. Sometimes this process can take considerable time, but with persistence you are likely to find a laboratory that is the right fit. Remember to explore all of your options and to consider laboratories in a variety of locations. Attending research talks and reading widely are two good ways to become familiar with relevant research, which is key to finding your niche. Remember to bring your lab notebook to the lab and to talks. Take notes when you are reading research papers. You never know when you will be inspired. If there is a reception after a talk, do not dash out of the room, but rather use the opportunity to get to know those attending. Be persistent. Try to attend at least one research talk a week and to read several research papers. Get outside of your comfort zone. See what is happening at local universities, institutions, and foundations. Start to meet researchers that are not just at your local university, deliberately undertaking to expand your network and ways of thinking.

Once you have found the right laboratory, now it is time to get started on your research project. The exercises at the end of each chapter of this book will help you to read the literature and to begin to formulate questions. Next, we will discuss your first weeks in a laboratory.

Summary (check off your achievements)

- Get a notebook for your research. _____
- Always be professional. _____
- Know your goals. _____
- Demonstrate that the lab is your first priority. _____
- Be persistent. _____
- Determine the email address you will use. _____
- Know and map out your schedule. _____
- Set aside 5–10 hours a week for reading relevant literature. _____

EXERCISES

1. This exercise is designed both to help you select a laboratory and to begin writing your thesis or research paper. You may find papers or journal articles to review by using the guidelines in this book, or they be handpicked and assigned. Reading five papers is a fair bit of work, but it's worth it. With every paper you read, you learn more about the research process. Reading research papers can be likened to visiting a museum in that fresh glimmers of knowledge and insight arise each time you view a painting or sculpture. Just as when comparing various artists, similarly when comparing various research teams, one finds that they employ vastly different styles.

Process these papers thoroughly, and answer the questions below. The first time that you do this exercise, it may take you a long time, but once you have repeated the process a few times you will find that it becomes much easier. Note that there are highlighted terms in each of the questions below. There are three main elements you should be looking for in a research paper:

1. **What's the question** that the researchers are exploring?
2. **Why is this an important question** that needed to be addressed?
3. How did the researchers solve the problem? In other words, what did the research team find that is **new**?

These are the same key elements that you need to address when writing up your own research papers. As you conduct this exercise, you will discover that these questions are answered more clearly in some research papers than in others. When writing up your own research papers, try to emulate the style of those authors who most successfully focus on the three key points above.

Paper 1 Title: _____

_____

What research question did the study address? _____

_____

_____

Why is the question important to address? _____

_____

_____

What was new about the study? How did it fill in gaps in the literature? _____

_____

_____

What are some of the limitations and future directions of the study? What ideas do you have for future studies? _____

_____

_____

Paper 2 Title: _____

_____

What research question did the study address? _____

_____

_____

Why is the question important to address? _____

_____

_____

What was new about the study? How did it fill in gaps? _____

_____

_____

What are some of the limitations and future directions of the study? What ideas do you have for future studies? _____

_____

_____

Paper 3 Title: _____

_____

What research question did the study address? _____

_____

_____

Why is the question important to address? _____

_____

_____

What was new about the study? How did it fill in gaps? _____

_____

_____

What are some of the limitations and future directions of the study? What ideas do you have for future studies? _____

_____

_____

Paper 4 Title: _____

_____

What research question did the study address? _____

_____

_____

Why is the question important to address? _____

_____

_____

What was new about the study? How did it fill in gaps? _____

_____

_____

What are some of the limitations and future directions of the study? What ideas do you have for future studies? _____

_____

_____

Paper 5 Title: _____

_____

What research question did the study address? _____

_____

_____

Why is the question important to address? _____

_____

_____

What was new about the study? How did it fill in gaps? _____

_____

_____

What are some of the limitations and future directions of the study? What ideas
do you have for future studies? _____

_____

_____

Summary of Exercise 1: Research demands lots of time, careful reading, writing, and critical analysis. Just imagine the time that goes into the research underlying one of these papers. If you are in the process of selecting a laboratory,
do you feel inspired and enthusiastic yet about any of the laboratories that you
might be interested in working in? If you are already working in a laboratory, the
exercises will help to focus you on developing interesting research questions
and writing up research papers. Whether you are a novice or a seasoned researcher, reading and reviewing research papers with an eye toward these three
key elements—(1) What's the question?, (2) Why is it an important question?, and
(3) What's new?—will assist you in dealing with the research process. You will
notice that I repeat this point throughout the guide, given its great importance.

Notes: _____

_____

_____

2. Imagine that you are preparing for your lab interview. List the questions
you intended to ask below. If you are in a class, you might even rehearse a mock
interview with your classmates. Are some of your questions related to research
papers that you read to prepare yourself for the interview?

1. _____

_____

2. _____

_____

3. _____

_____

4. _____

_____

5. _____

_____

3. Imagine that you are starting a position in a new laboratory. Fill in your time availabilities (with an X) below. Bring a copy of the filled-in form to your interview.

Name: _____

Date: _____

Email address: _____

Person/no. to contact in emergency: _____

Start date: _____

Notes: _____

_____

_____

	Mon.	Tues.	Wed.	Thurs.	Fri.	Sat.	Sun.
9							
10							
11							
12							
1							
2							
3							
4							
5							
6							

4. List ten reasons why you think that the laboratory you are planning to work in or are currently working in is doing important research. Why might a parent or educator want to participate in a research study with his or her infant or young child (or why might a teen want to take part)? If you are taking a course, your professor may suggest labs for you to consider.

1. _____

   _____

2. To learn more and understand how his or her child develops!

   _____

3. _____

   _____

4. _____

   _____

5. _____

   _____

6. For social reasons—maybe he or she wants to meet other parents

   and get out of the house.

7. _____

   _____

8. _____

   _____

9. _____

   _____

10. _____

    _____

5. **Be creative with your resources.** If you had only $3.50 to run an entire research study involving 20 children, how would you motivate the parents and families to participate? List some ways below.

1. _____

_____

_____

2. _____

_____

_____

3. I would offer a diploma for the children and a free summary of the

results of the research online. _____

_____

4. _____

_____

_____

5. _____

_____

_____

6. I would organize an educational event for the families and children,

charge $10 to participate, but then offer an entry-free coupon to

those families that volunteer to participate in my research project!

7. I would use the $3.50 for postage and then mail out requests for local

community organizations to sponsor the study. _____

_____

6. **Finding solutions and strategies.** If you had $8 (total) to run a longitudinal research study involving sixteen 12-year-old boys, in six sessions of 30 minutes each, how would you convince the boys to participate? List your answers below.

1. _____

_____

2. _____

_____

3. *I would let them choose among several inexpensive gifts. . . .*

_____

4. _____

_____

CHAPTER 2

Your First Days and Weeks in the Laboratory

What should I expect during my first days and weeks in a laboratory?

The answer depends on the specific laboratory where you are working. In most laboratories, you should expect to get a tour of the lab, a brief description of ongoing research studies, and a review of the rules and regulations governing the laboratory. Most likely, the laboratory that you have chosen will have clear protocols and guidelines in place. If not, you might begin working on developing a more optimal research culture by helping to create appropriate protocols. What are the procedures for entering the laboratory and for locking it when closing? How will you get the keys (if at all)? What are the hours of operation? Speak with prior or current lab members to find out about the relevant guidelines. Contacting prior lab members is a great way to find out what worked and to obtain information that perhaps even your mentor does not have.

Where are research papers filed? Are there passwords on the computers? Where are these stored? Where are the lab's promotional materials stored? What are the procedures and protocols for answering the phone? Where is the form for signing out and signing in equipment? What are the procedures for logging one's working hours and activities? What are the emergency and safety procedures? Where is the first-aid kit?

The institutional review board: Start with the basics.

This is also the time to become familiar with institutional review boards (IRB), ethical committees and guidelines, and any courses required before you can begin recruiting and working with infants and children. The specific guidelines naturally depend on your particular laboratory, institute, or university. In general, research conducted with human subjects must be reviewed and approved by an external board in order to protect the rights of the participants. This approval process must be completed before you begin testing anyone. One of the best ways to get your proposals for research approved is to plan ahead and get to know and understand your local IRB. In most cases, there will be an IRB on your campus. Sometimes these boards have open information sessions on conducting research and completing the complex forms often involved with research on humans.

How might I learn more about the IRB protocols and procedures?

One of the best ways to learn is to observe what people working in the laboratory have done before you. Does your laboratory have a website? Have you studied it thoroughly? In most cases, you are not the first student or researcher to be involved with the laboratory. Ask to read the current protocols and the IRB notices relating to the laboratory issued over the past 5 years. This process should give you some sense of how your particular laboratory develops and deals with research proposals. In the process, you may also learn how the laboratory is itself organized.

Before initiating your research, you may need to demonstrate that you are familiar with the rules and regulations governing your lab's human subject research. Many universities and research institutions are members of the Collaborative Institutional Training Initiative, known as CITI. Visit the IRB website of your university or institute, where their guidelines should be available. At my current university the guidelines are provided online as several clear steps, one of which initially is for all key personnel to complete the CITI Training Program.

For a summary of the program, visit *www.citiprogram.org.* "The CITI Program is a subscription service providing research ethics education to all members of the research community. To participate fully, learners must be affiliated with a CITI participating organization." When you have completed the program, you will need to print out a certificate to keep on file listing the IRB protocols and perhaps also the laboratory that you are working in. In many cases, students interested in working in my laboratory have already taken the CITI course as part of a basic research methods course. If this is the case for you, check that you have completed all the required modules and, if so, reprint your certificate, to be kept on file. You should check with the laboratory that you are working in for specific requirements.

 Think ahead. If you are planning a new study, you might have to submit a new protocol if it is not covered under the preexisting one in the laboratory that you are working in. The review process might take *up to 6 months* or even longer.

As you learn about IRBs, you might also wish to learn more about the First Amendment, the Freedom of Information Act, and perhaps even get more familiar with copyright and intellectual property laws in the United States (or whichever country you are working in). A basic understanding of the law is essential for being an effective and successful researcher and scholar.

I'm just getting started. Do I really need to know about IRB protocols?

You most likely do not have to begin writing your IRB protocols on your first day in the lab, but I think it is a good idea to have a sense of what you will need to do before you begin your research. *Having a plan* will help you to develop a research and time management strategy (as will be further elaborated in later chapters).

Before you begin your research study, you will need to have it approved by the IRB. The IRB proposal described later provides a summary of the research to be conducted as well as the procedures the research team deems necessary for obtaining informed consent and the various general protocols. A great deal of preparation is involved in conducting research with infants and children. During your first weeks in the laboratory, get a sense of what is involved and plan ahead. You may also want to ask the IRB or the department that you are working within whether samples are available for you. Generally, researchers are happy to share their expertise and protocols.

Do you have examples?

Here I provide an example of an IRB protocol from my own lab that can be used as a guide as you develop your own. Note that the guidelines may differ for your individual school or institution. Sometimes IRB proposals are written for a very specific project, and at other times such proposals are intended to cover a series of related studies.

Try to write in a clear and direct manner. Your proposal should be accessible and free of jargon. Remember that members of the IRB may be drawn from a variety of departments or academic fields. Also keep in mind that they may be reading dozens of proposals at any given time. Enable them to finish reviewing your proposal promptly simply because it was clearly written.

Project: Social Monitoring

1. **Purpose of Research:** The purpose of our study is to establish the development and function of joint attention/social monitoring skills in the child's first year. [**Note:** Here we used a general topic so that several studies could be conducted under this protocol.]

   Hypotheses: By as early as 3–4 months of age, infants will show sensitivity to joint attention skills and use these cues to learn.

   Research Design: Infants will be tested between 2 and 24 months. Depending on the given study, we will assess infants for 1–5 minutes as they interact with people and objects. [**Note:** We used a broad age range for this general proposal, which gave us some flexibility when testing infants.]

2. **Subject Recruitment and Selection Criteria:** Participants will be recruited via telephone, email, and in person. We will actively recruit around the New York City area. We will contact places such as day cares, schools, after-school programs, local magazines, parenting sites, and other places where children gather. In addition, we will use contact information from our database. The lab's database consists of children whose parents have expressed an interest in having their children participate in developmental research and have agreed to have their contact information stored in our database. Recruitment methods for the database have been described in a separate HRPP proposal titled *Database Recruitment (Protocol #)*. Selection criteria for children require that they are typically developing, with an age ranging from newborns to 17 years of age. Male and female participants will be recruited equally. Given New York City's high rate of racial

and ethnic diversity, we expect that our sample will reflect that diversity in similar percentages. [**Note:** This laboratory has a separate IRB for recruitment. This means that even if a particular study is not being conducted, infants and children may still be recruited.]

3. **Description of the Procedures:** Infants will engage with their caregiver or a stranger and an object for 1 to 3 minutes in a joint attention or non-joint attention context. Infants will then be presented with various objects, and their visual preference toward these objects will be assessed. Caregivers will be seated behind the participants, and there will be no distractions such as noise or objects in the surrounding area. Participants will receive a small gift of appreciation for participating in the study. Infant/child participants will receive a small gift such as a T-shirt, a box of crayons, a coloring book, or a toy for participating. Participants will receive the gift even if they have not completed the study (e.g., if they have chosen to stop testing at any given time).

4. **Potential Harms or Benefits:** Our research will pose no potential harm to participants beyond minimal risks involved in ordinary human interaction. Procedures and length of stimulus presentation will vary among studies and will be adjusted to complement the infant/child participant's attention span. Breaks will be given to participants if they become fussy, and the procedure will be discontinued if they do not become calm after the break. There are no potential benefits to the infants or their guardian. The scientific community may benefit from our contribution. Results will also help us to determine the social cues that help infants learn. We are not trained to diagnose developmental disorders and will not use our data to diagnose participants. We will clarify this for legal guardians of the child participants and to the adult participants in the recruiting process and within the Consent Form.

5. **Methods by Which Confidentiality will be Protected:** Confidentiality will be ensured by storing data without names or identifying information. Each participant will be given an identification code, and the data will be stored with this code only. The code will consist of nine symbols. The first four symbols will be numeric and will represent the order in which we were given permission to add the child into the database. The next symbol will be either an M or an F and will distinguish male and female participants. The next two symbols will be numeric and represent the month in which the participant was born. The last two symbols will be numeric and will represent the year in which the participant was born. Therefore, if the first participant recruited is a girl born in February of 2008, her code will be: 0001F0208. The data will be stored in a locked file cabinet in a locked office for a minimum of 3 years.

6. **Debriefing Procedures**: Our research will not include deception. We will explain to participants that we are not qualified to determine whether a child might show any signs of atypical development. If parents raise any concerns about their infant/child's development to us, we will clearly state that we are unable to provide any sort of advice or diagnosis. We will advise parents that if they have any concerns that they should consult their pediatrician.

7. **Oral and Written Consent Procedures**: Infant/child's legal guardian (or authorized caregiver) will be briefed verbally concerning what participation entails for both their child and themselves. They will then be given the opportunity to ask questions and will be presented with a Consent Form for the child participant and/or themselves. Additionally, since all testing will be videotaped, in order to participate, adult participants and the legal guardians of the child participants will have to sign our Video Consent Form. Furthermore, some adult participants will be presented with a Photograph Consent Form. Once all of their questions have been answered to their satisfaction, and it is clear that legal guardians understand the procedures, and granted permission of their participation, we will begin the study. In some instances the legal guardian may express to have a caregiver (e.g., a nanny or a grandparent) bring the child in for the study. In these cases, we will mail the Consent Form, the Video Consent Form, and the Authorization of Caregiver Other than Legal Guardians Form to the legal guardian. The legal guardian must then mail all completed and signed forms to our lab. We will not schedule a test date with the child until these forms are received. If someone other than a legal guardian brings a child for testing unexpectedly, the child will not be tested.

8. **Other Pertinent Information**: Not applicable.

9. **References**: Not applicable.

    Note: Often the IRB will ask for revisions. In such cases it is best to meet with the IRB in person so that you fully understand their concerns and can address these effectively.

May I start data collection tomorrow?

Have you had your project approved by the IRB? If not, now is the time to submit your proposal to the IRB and begin to develop strategies for recruitment. On pages 37–42 I provide another example of IRB forms

that may guide you and give you ideas as you develop your own protocols. Be sure also to check with your supervisor to see if your research
study can be covered under an existing umbrella or amended research
protocol. If your proposal is under review, you might want to run a
mock study with your lab mates as participants. You might even take a
video of the proposed procedure and show it during a lab meeting. Your
lab mates and mentor could then provide feedback.

That proposal was very detailed. When do I have to write one?

At this stage you may not have to develop your own IRB protocols, but
it is a good idea to know what is involved in writing your IRB protocols
so that you can plan and manage your time effectively. Your mentor will
likely give you more details about when to submit your IRB proposal
or whether your study is already covered under an existing protocol.
Remember that in the preceding chapter I indicated that research with
infants and children is very time-consuming. You will have to do some
strategic planning. You may also start investigating how currently
active IRB protocols in your laboratory may be amended. The process
of changing or adding to an active protocol is often much simpler than
submitting a brand-new protocol.

I have read through all the IRB forms. Now what?

Now is also a great time to return to Chapter 1, to the exercises in the
back of that chapter, and to continue reading research papers in the
lab that you are working in or research papers that have been recommended to you by the lab director. Later chapters in the book provide
guidelines on how to select research papers if you are not sure where
to begin.

Do I need funding for research?

When conducting research you often have limited financial or other
resources and need to find fundraising solutions to get your research
done. Perhaps you would like to pursue research during the summer
months as well or to attend a conference in Singapore next year. Most

likely, you would need additional funding for that. Perhaps you would like to provide the children with a special gift or custom coloring book for participating in your research study but you lack the financial resources to pay for it on your own. Sometimes you need to be especially creative to get your research fully done. As you develop your research skills, try to find effective solutions for the problems that you encounter along the way. You might ask your mentor about possible fundraising events or consider various grant opportunities for students that are available from many sources. Research grants are often available through such public sources as the National Science Foundation (NSF) or the National Institutes of Health (NIH). There are also many international grants and other funding opportunities available. Many specialized organizations offer student travel awards or undergraduate research awards that enable you to attend conferences or conduct some of your research. For instance, this summer one of the undergraduates in my laboratory obtained funding through a travel award to attend the International Conference on Infant Studies. To be considered for the grant, she needed to be the primary author of an abstract submitted to the conference and to write two required essays. Even more crucially, she needed to be *made aware* of this opportunity. Let your mentors know if you are seeking special funding and join professional organizations and email lists for timely communications about upcoming grants. You might even want to contact past recipients of special awards or grants in the field directly for their advice on how to best present your application and credentials.

Many universities also offer internal funding for research projects. The key to adequately funding your research often involves having a great idea and then planning ahead. To obtain a grant for your research, begin your planning at least 12 months in advance of your needs. This will give you sufficient time to fill out the necessary forms, develop your ideas, write a research proposal, and obtain any needed reference letters. Most likely, your mentor and those supporting your application will need at least 8 weeks to plan, prepare, and send their reference letters off to grant agencies. Your university or academic advisor may be able to guide you. Most grants have specific deadlines. If a grant's deadline is 5:00 P.M. on October 1 and you discovered the grant only a week earlier, most likely you will need to wait an additional year to apply. Get a listing of grant deadlines from organizations in your field or your academic advisor. Set yourself apart from others possibly even enabling by planning ahead. Research at the more advanced stages almost always involves grant funding. Grant funding may also be helpful to support your work and research during the summer months. It may allow you to spend time in a laboratory abroad and thereby providing opportunities to learn new skills while broadening the experience.

Even if you do not need grant funding for your study, it is never too early to get involved in the grant writing process if you are considering a career that involves research. As a graduate student, I often helped out with grants by proofreading, counting pages, collating supporting materials and otherwise assisting them. Through that process I learned a great deal about the stamina, dedication, and preparation needed to write and obtain grants. My mentor also shared grant reviews with me whenever they came in, whether these reviews were negative or positive. Seeing these critical reviews helped me develop my own research skills. With my mentor's input, I learned how to cope with rejection early in my career. This is an important part of the research process. Of course, I found it devastating to think that I could read a grant description so many times, count so many pages, and simply work so hard and yet not be successful. However, learning to deal with rejection can make you a more passionate and determined researcher and grant application writer. Rejection also makes you appreciate your successes. Having the opportunity to share in the grant preparation experience with your mentor can be instrumental to your eventual success. The take-home message here is to try to get involved with as many aspects of research as possible even if, at the time, they do not seem 100% relevant. The research process does not end at 5:00 P.M. or when a research paper is submitted to a journal. Get involved in *all* aspects of research early on, from organizing the lab, to public relations and outreach, to grant writing and reviewing research papers.

Summary (check off your achievements)

- Learn about your local IRB. _____
- Help to further develop or learn about your lab's operating guidelines. _____
- Closely examine the existing IRB protocols. _____
- Join relevant professional organizations. _____
- Read funded grant proposals. _____
- Learn all about diverse funding opportunities. _____
- Create a chart detailing deadlines for upcoming grants. _____

EXERCISES

1. Read about the Code of Federal Regulations at *www.hhs.gov/ohrp/ policy/ohrpregulations.pdf.* Also read about how the typical IRB is formed and why at *www.hhs.gov/ohrp/assurances/irb/index.html.* In your view, what are the advantages and disadvantages of forming an IRB? Please explain each one.

_____

_____

_____

_____

_____

_____

_____

_____

_____

_____

2. Visit the following websites that focus on ethics, and discuss some possible unforeseen consequences of research. How might you avoid harm to participants in research? Can you provide examples?

American Psychological Association
www.apa.org/ethics/code

The Society for Research in Child Development
www.srcd.org/about-us/ethical-standards-research

European Commission on Research
http://ec.europa.eu/research/index.cfm

Canadian Code of Conduct for Research Involving Humans
www.ethics.ubc.ca/code

Office for Human Research Protections
www.hhs.gov/ohrp
"OHRP [Office for Human Research Protections] works to ensure that human subjects outside of the United States who participate in research projects conducted or funded by DHHS [U.S. Department of Health and Human Services] receive the same level of protections as research participants inside the United States. To that end, the OHRP International

Activities program offers consultation services, disseminates pertinent reports, and provides research ethics training" (*www.hhs.gov/ohrp/ international/index.html*).

Ethical Issues in Research with Children & Research Involving Persons at Risk for Impaired Decision National Institutes of Health *http://videocast.nih.gov/summary.asp?live=7867&bhcp=1*

Notes for discussion: _____

_____

_____

_____

_____

_____

_____

_____

3. Read "Ethical Standards in Research" at *www.srcd.org/about-us/ ethical-standards-research*. In your view, what are some fair incentives for participating in research?

_____

_____

_____

_____

_____

_____

_____

_____

_____

_____

Theoretically, would you let your own child participate in a research study? Why or why not? Based on your response, what should researchers bear in mind?

_____

_____

_____

_____

_____

_____

If your child had a disability, would you let him or her participate in research? Why or why not? _____

_____

_____

_____

_____

_____

4. Read "How Many Scientists Fabricate?" at *www.plosone.org/article/ info%3Adoi%2F10.1371%2Fjournal.pone.0005738*, or conduct an Internet search for "data fabrication" and related terms.

What would you do if you suspected that data fraud was being perpetrated on a project you were involved in? Why? _____

_____

_____

_____

_____

_____

_____

In your opinion, what should happen to scientists who fabricate data? _____

_____

_____

_____

_____

_____

_____

PARENT AND EDUCATOR EMAIL SCRIPT

Project Title: Database

Hello Educators and Parents,

We are writing on behalf of the _____ Laboratory at [your school], where we study social development, learning, cognition, and communication in early development.

We are eager to hear from educators and parents of children from birth to 10 years of age who would like to learn more about early development. We would also like to introduce our new website, _____.*com*, which provides an overview of our ongoing research studies in child development as well as past publications, local schools, and relevant resources in New York City.

Our research is widely published and is often of interest to parents, educators, and the media. To learn more, please visit our website provided above, call us at 212-xxx-xxxx, or send an email to [email address]. In addition, we invite you to visit our research facility or have us visit your school, parents' group, or organization.

We look forward to hearing from you!

Sincerely,
[name of your laboratory]

Director, [name], PhD
Professor of Psychology, [school name]
[school address]
[blog/website]

Reprinted with permission from Wesleyan University.

PARENT CONSENT FORM

Background

You are being asked to have your child participate in a research study that examines how children use social cues to learn about their environment. This experiment is under the supervision of Dr. _____, Director of [name of college's/university's] _____ Laboratory.

Participation in this study is voluntary, and refusal to participate will involve no penalty or loss of benefits to which you are entitled.

Procedures

Your child is being asked to participate in a study of social cognition in infancy. Your infant/child will sit on your lap and interact with an adult experimenter who will show your infant various objects while varying social cues. The testing procedure, which is noninvasive, will depend on the age of your child. If your baby becomes fussy for more than 45 consecutive seconds, we will conclude that he or she does not consent to participating and we will end the experiment. You are free to stop testing at any time without penalty or loss of benefits. Your child will receive a small gift such as a T-shirt or book for participating in the study. Your child will receive the gift even if he or she does not complete the procedure.

Risks and/or Discomforts

There are no known risks associated with participation in this study. Some infants may get fussy during the procedure. If this happens, your infant can take a short break before proceeding. If taking a break is not enough to calm your infant, the procedure can be stopped at any time.

Benefits

There are no direct benefits.

Your Rights as a Research Participant

You have rights as the legal guardian of a research volunteer. Taking part in this study is voluntary. If your infant/child expresses an unwillingness to participate through behavior such as fussing for more than 45 consecutive seconds, the study will be ended. If you have questions about your legal rights as the legal guardian of a research volunteer, call or write:

(continued)

Name of School
Human Research Protection Program (HRPP)
Address
Room Number
Phone Number / Fax Number

Privacy and Confidentiality

The experimenters will video record the procedure with your permission. You will be given a separate form to indicate your permission. The procedure is video recorded so that the data can be analyzed at a later time.

No identifying information will be stored with the video images. Likewise, any data from your child will be stored without any identifying information. The recordings and data will be stored in a secure locked location. Only the research team will know that you participated in the study. The researcher is mandated to report to the proper authorities suspected child abuse.

Contact Information

If you have questions about the study, you can contact Dr. _____ at 212-xxx-xxxx. He/she is located at [school name and address]. You should contact the [school name] HRPP Office at 212-xxx-xxxx, if you have questions regarding your rights or your child's rights as a subject or if you feel you have been harmed as a result of you or your child's participation in this research.

Signatures

I have read (or have had read to me) the contents of this consent form and have been encouraged to ask questions. I have received answers to my questions. I voluntarily give my consent to have my child participate in this study. I have received (or will receive) a copy of this form for my records and future reference.

Participant's Name: _____ Participant's Birth Date: _____

Parent's or Guardian's Name: _____

Signature: _____ Date: _____

Researcher's Name: _____

Signature: _____ Date: _____

VIDEO RECORDING RELEASE CONSENT FORM

Protocol Title: Social Monitoring

As part of this project, a videotape recording will be made of your child's participation in this research project. This will allow us to carefully analyze your child's behavior during the testing. We sometimes also will use the videotaped images and/or pictures to educate the public and the scientific community about our results. Please indicate below the uses of these videotapes and/or pictures for which you are willing to consent. This is completely voluntary, and you will not be penalized for choosing not to permit some uses. None of the videotapes and/or pictures will identify you or your child personally.

1. The videos and/or pictures can be studied by the research team for use in the research project. _____ Initials

2. The videos and/or pictures can be shown at meetings of scientists interested in the study of child development. _____ Initials

3. The videos and/or pictures can be shown in classrooms to students. _____ Initials

4. The videos and/or pictures can be shown in public presentations to nonscientific groups. _____ Initials

5. The videos and/or pictures can be shown on television. _____ Initials

6. The videos and/or pictures may be used in media such as, but not limited to, PowerPoint presentations, websites, booklets, DVDs, and books. _____ Initials

You have read the above description and give your consent for the use of videotapes as indicated above.

Participant's Name: _____ Participant's Birth Date: _____

Legal Guardian's Name: _____

Signature: _____ Date: _____

PHOTO RELEASE CONSENT FORM

Protocol Title: Social Monitoring

As part of a research project, photographs will be taken of you and edited in Photoshop. At some point we may want to use your pictures as stimuli for studies in our lab. YOU ARE **NOT** REQUIRED TO ALLOW YOUR PHOTOS TO BE USED AS STUDY STIMULI. We sometimes also will use the pictures to educate the public and the scientific community about our results. Please indicate below the uses of these pictures for which you are willing to consent. This is completely voluntary, and you will not be penalized for choosing not to permit some uses. None of the pictures will identify you personally.

1. The pictures can be used by the research team for the research project. _____
   Initials

2. The pictures can be shown at meetings of scientists interested in the study of infant–child development. _____Initials

3. The pictures can be shown in classrooms to students. _____ Initials

4. The pictures can be shown in public presentations to on-scientific groups. _____
   Initials

5. The pictures can be shown on television. _____ Initials

6. The pictures can be used in media such as, but not limited to, PowerPoint presentations, websites, booklets, DVDs, and books. _____ Initials

You have read the above description and give your consent for the use of photographs as indicated above.

Participant's Name: _____ Participant's Birth Date: _____

Legal Guardian's Name: _____

Signature: _____ Date: _____

CAREGIVER OTHER THAN LEGAL GUARDIAN AUTHORIZATION FORM

Researcher: Dr. _____

Protocol Title: Social Monitoring

I, _____ , the legal guardian of _____ ,
am aware of and consenting to having my child participate in a research study of
children's social development at the Infancy Research Laboratory at [school name]
or at his/her school, _____ .

I give my consent to have my authorized caregiver bring my child to and from the
laboratory and observe my child's participation in the study. The authorized caregiver
understands that if he or she is uncomfortable with the experimental procedure, he
or she may stop the process at any time and still receive a gift for my child.

Participant's Name: _____ Participant's Birth Date: _____

Parent's or Guardian's Name: _____

Signature: _____ Date: _____

Caretaker's Name: _____

Caretaker's Relationship to the Participating Child (e.g., nanny or grandparent): _____

_____

CHAPTER 3

Managing Your Time

You likely realize by now that research takes more time than you expected. It is important to set aside enough time for research and to develop strategies to work efficiently. You need to have a clear head to do research efficiently. Therefore, if you go and party the night before you are to be in the laboratory, there is a good chance that you will not write and think very well the next day. You need to set your priorities. Also remember that it is not the number of hours that counts, but your measurable productivity and output. Use your time wisely. If you write best in the morning, dedicate that time to writing. Having a routine also helps. For instance, I seem to get my best writing done between 7:30 A.M. and 11:00 A.M. In the evening, I like to work on lab-related social media or less demanding tasks. If you are planning to write in the morning, try not to check your emails or turn on the television before you begin, but rather immediately get to work. You might then work on recruiting participants at around 1 P.M. to 3 P.M. each day. On the other hand, if you are a night owl, you might write at 10 P.M. to 1 A.M. and save your afternoons for less demanding tasks.

Working effectively with guidelines

Now, as a first priority, you want to become familiar with the guidelines of the research laboratory that you are working in so as to begin developing a plan for your research and scheduling. Even in the most effficently run laboratories, problems can arise. In many cases, these problems reflect a lack of communication and/or a lack of documentation regarding the expectations and goals of the particular researchers working there. In order to keep in good standing in a research laboratory, you need to keep up with your work and timelines. One way to do this is by developing a time management strategy that is agreed upon with your lab supervisor or mentor. Some basic forms are provided at the end of this chapter that should help you with the task of time management.

Remember, you can always update a contract and a timeline, but persistent failure to complete tasks or projects on time can result in your being asked to leave the laboratory. A laboratory often has a different feel from a typical company, but the rules observed are basically the same. If you and your mentor/supervisor have agreed on specified working hours each week, you are expected not to change these hours without discussing the matter with your mentor or supervisor in advance. As a rule of thumb, think of your work in the research laboratory in much the same terms as you would full-time employment in any law firm, business establishment, or hospital.

> *Doing a PhD on your own can be a lonely undertaking; so, you have to fight the natural tendency that most graduate students have of working from home!*

This advice holds true whatever your stage of research. Be sure to remain active and be seen frequently in the lab. Using a Lab Sign-In Sheet like the one on page 60 is a great way to keep track of your progress in the laboratory.

> *I meet graduate students once a week for a meeting. They have half-an-hour to talk about anything they want. Then they know that I might be busy and they need to see if they can meet with me at other times. I always use the PhD by publication route. There are two ways you can be awarded a PhD in the UK. One is compiling a dissertation. The other is via publication. This pathway means that you need to publish a minimum of three articles and then write an introduction, explaining the overarching issues that link the papers, and then a discussion chapter. This way the student has a good vita by the time they finish, so there is a higher chance that they get a job!"*
> —Dr. Vincent Reid, Professor, Lancaster University

I have met various "professional graduate students" over the years. A lack of communication with a mentor or a lack of planning in general may result in a student's spending many extra years in graduate school.

Remember that planning adequately is an important cornerstone of being a successful developmental researcher (as well as achieving success in many career choices). If you are trying to graduate from a program or complete a project, then you should definitely consider time management strategies.

Be mindful. Be planful.
—Dr. Roseanne Flores, Associate Professor, Hunter College

If you are writing a large thesis, perhaps it is because your project is a portion of a larger-scale project that will be published in its entirety eventually, perhaps as a monograph or book. You might be conducting a longitudinal study, asking a question such as "Do positive facial expressions in newborn infants predict peer relations in the first grade?" If this is your overarching research question and you have only 18 months of funding, you may want to write a dissertation that focuses on the first phase of the project. Perhaps you could follow up later on these infants after you have defended your thesis. Thinking that you have to cover *everything* in your thesis is a common misconception often observable in conscientious students. Always keep in mind that your thesis is most likely not the last scholarly project that you will ever undertake. Even if it *is* your final research project, you will probably want to have lasting positive memories of the experience. Your thesis or dissertation represents a unique opportunity to learn and to give yourself the chance to plan, manage your time, think critically, defend your ideas and findings, and *complete* a project. If your project is too grand in its aspirations, you may not even get to the oral defense stage of it. This advice is especially critical for honors students who need to complete their projects in order to graduate on time.

Plan ahead! Know what statistical tests you are going to use before starting data acquisition, and design your study accordingly. Calculate the resources that will be required realistically (subjects, lab space, time, etc.).
—Dr. Stefanie Hoehl, Assistant Professor, Heidelberg University

How long will it take me to write?

Do you love to write? Perhaps writing comes naturally to you, and you will write your thesis over the course of a couple of long days. On the other hand, you may find writing to be a highly painful activity. In this case, perhaps you end up writing for 1–2 hours a day over the course of 2–3 weeks. Your response to this question depends largely on your own strengths and weaknesses and will likely influence how long it takes you to complete the task. You must find your own routine and write as much as possible, "to keep in shape." To use the exercise metaphor, writing is much like doing push-ups (in that you must do them almost every day to keep in shape!). I have met many researchers who love to write and find it naturally rewarding. It is as if (shifting again to the athletic realm) they were born with amazing muscle tone or some innate athletic abilities. It is important to keep in mind that even Olympic athletes must practice and perform daily. I personally find doing push-ups far more rewarding than writing. If you are like me, you might want to consider the specific setting in which you are doing your research and writing. Finding the right environment to work in can help you to perform more optimally. You need to try to maximize your productivity by finding or creating your own optimal environment for writing. With experience, you will learn about the work settings in which you function and perform best. As you develop that experience, begin to develop routines for your writing and research activities. This will help you to monitor and predict how long it should take you to write your thesis or to develop a proposal. If you are not satisfied with the ongoing result, it is important to modify your routine accordingly.

When I was a student, my mentor would insist that I write for 3 hours a day before noon. He would not speak to me or answer any email from me during this time (it was probably his writing time too!). He said that even if I just sat there for 3 hours it was okay but that I just had to learn to develop a routine. Nearly 20 years later, this experience still drives me. When I do not feel like writing, I force myself to do so by sitting in front of the computer. Whether I produced 10 words or 10 pages, I developed a routine to see important projects through. In the next chapter, we will discuss the importance of developing a culture of research. Immersing yourself in the right culture can have a dramatic effect on your productivity and performance. Spend time around those who keep busy writing (as opposed to those more inclined to just sit in the lab discussing matters or thinking about writing) and draw inspiration from their example through interaction with them. Calculate the time it will take you to write your proposal, and if that calculation is not acceptable, change your routine or environment. Discuss solutions and strategies with your mentor. You are the only one with the power to change the situation. Do not underestimate the time it takes to plan your strategy, write your proposal, and conduct your research.

How can I determine how long it will take to recruit participants?

As you are thinking about your proposal and a time management plan for your research study, you will want to think about how you might recruit participants and how long this will take. In part, this will depend on your skills, the location, and your effort. The most critical element is certainly your "effort." Twenty years of experience in locations ranging from Boston to Atlanta, from Leipzig, Germany, to New York City, taught me that effort is the most critical element of recruiting children. It does not matter whether only one child is born at the hospital or 30 children in the same day. It does not matter whether you encounter only one child at the park or 50 children playing outside. It does not matter whether a well-established laboratory or a well-known university stands behind your efforts. It should not matter if you offer children a sticker for participating or a $20 silkscreen printed T-shirt. The real key is caring passionately about what you do, being able to communicate it and why it is important to parents, and simply getting to it (i.e., exerting sufficient effort). If you care about what you are doing, parents and caregivers will sense that and likely be happy and honored to participate. If you are undertaking a thesis or project merely in order to graduate with "honors" or just because your boyfriend or girlfriend is doing it, potential participants will sense that too. Most likely this will result in more time spent in both recruiting your participants and completing your research project. Be sure that you are doing research for all the right reasons, and rapid success is much more likely to come your way. Your drive will set you apart and help you to complete your project efficiently. However, you might not be able to work a full-time job, take a full course load, and still complete a research project efficiently and on time. Rather, you may need to prioritize your goals.

Drive helps get the job done.

One mild summer day, two research assistants of mine complained that they were able to recruit only two participants in New York City. I asked them to meet with me in Central Park at 4:00 P.M. so that we could discuss their progress. As I was approaching them in the park, I saw them sitting on a bench staring at the walkway as they were waiting for me. Since dozens of babies were being strolled by and scores of children were running about in the playground just 10 feet away, why weren't they actively engaged in recruiting potential participants? One of the assistants later dubbed me her "lucky charm"—as it seemed that her success increased 20-fold when I was standing by her and pointing out each parent and child who walked by! You need drive and persistence to get your research done. If you do not feel comfortable approaching people or this process is not allowable under your IRB protocols, then set up a situation in which parents approach *you*. You must be active and creative when recruiting participants for your study or when getting to know people in the community. Hold events such as lab tours, research-based park events, holiday parties, or reading events at local libraries or the park (a subject further explored in Chapter 6).

As a rule of thumb, if you are unable to recruit one to three participants an hour, think about why. Are you passionate about your project? If the answer is "yes" and you have exhausted all the possibilities for recruitment, immediately consult with your mentor. If your mentor is like me, he or she will want to see and hear about the methods you have used to achieve your recruiting goals. He or she will want to see the flyers and social media tactics that you are using; will want to know how many parents you approached or contacted and how many agreed to participate in your research; and may even want to pretend he or she is a parent and see and hear your routine to help you make improvements. Also keep in mind that if 10 parents are interested in your study, you can generally expect only about 5 to be available (given their other commitments) and among those only 2 or 3 ultimately to participate. The numbers may also depend on your laboratory's reputation and location, of course, so get a sense from your mentor or senior researchers in the lab. In planning your project and managing your time, you will want to calculate everything from the time it will take to develop and print flyers, to the time it will take to organize networking events, to call parents to remind them about their visit to the laboratory, and of course the time it will take to write a summary of your research and share it with the parents.

You will want to critically analyze your problem in order to find solutions. If you were in direct contact with 15 parents and only 3 accepted your invitation to participate in research (for a noninvasive study), you may not be using an optimal script or conveying why the research is important or why it is worth their time (e.g., they will learn about their child's development, have a fun experience, meet other parents, or whatever the case might be). If, on the other hand, you were in direct contact with only three potential participants but all three accepted your invitation, you may not be optimizing your recruitment location and promotional possibilities but are probably pretty passionate about your study. Try to maximize your time management by being strategic about when, where, and how you recruit participants (e.g., no recruiting in parks on rainy days). If parents or potential participants are not accepting your invitation, take a step back and ask yourself why. Learn from the success of others in the laboratory or in other labs. Also remember that sometimes it is easier to convince parents to visit the laboratory when they can make an afternoon of it (and participate in more than one study or some parent education event), as opposed to visiting the laboratory for only a 3- to 5-minute study. Think strategically. Although this example pertains mainly to recruiting infants, the same principles apply regardless of the subject's age.

It is your responsibility to calculate how long it will take to recruit an adequate number of participants for your study. Use the time management guide in the back of this chapter to help you to plan. In addition, you will need to assume that some children will not make it into the laboratory and that therefore you will have to exclude some originally anticipated data from your final sample. For that reason, plan to test at least 10–15% more children than you will need in your final sample. It is very common for students to come to my office and say "I'm so happy! The study is done. I'm finished!" because they have tested the targeted 12 or 20 children in a group. However, sometimes they end up having to get back out there and collect more data. Sometimes a data point must be removed because of experimental error, or sometimes results show marginal significance level. In any case, research is usually not "finished" just because data collection is judged to be complete. Data collection is more likely to be completed effectively when you deliberately overestimate your required sample size.

How long will it take me to code participants?

Only you know the answer to this question. In part, this varies as a function of the number of your dependent measures. You want to address your question in the most precise way possible, and there should be a solid rationale for every behavior that you code. Less is often more. That said, sometimes it takes only 2–3 minutes to test a baby or child and then 1–5 hours to code the child's behavior. One way to assess how long it will take to code is to start coding as soon as you begin testing.

In that way you can assess how your results are coming along as the study progresses, and you will know exactly how long it is taking to code a child. It is important to not underestimate the amount of time it will take you to code the data, enter it into spreadsheets, and then analyze it. You can project how many hours it will take to code based on your experience with the first several participants.

Be sure also to schedule in time for unanticipated "disasters." If you are working on an honors project and have a preset deadline to meet in order to graduate, plan to complete your data collection 3–5+ weeks before the end of the semester. This allows you time to work on your presentations and to write up and submit your research to a journal. It also gives you peace of mind that your mentor will have time to read your thesis and provide critical feedback before your oral defense. You will likely need time to revise your "final" product based on feedback from your mentor and lab members. Also remember that children are often sick and you may end up becoming sick too. Try to stay healthy and think positively, but also plan ahead. If you will require testing 5 children a week to "stay on schedule" and defend your thesis on time, then aim to test 8–10 children a week.

Plan to give a mock defense of your thesis or dissertation about 3 weeks before the actual defense. Check with your mentor first, of course. Successful communication with your mentor is a crucial part of successful research. This leaves you 1 week to make revisions and another week for an additional practice talk. The week before your defense is not the time to be testing your final participants or figuring out what behaviors you will code. Develop a time management regimen early on and stick with it. Develop daily goals, weekly goals, and long-term goals. Check that you have met these goals each day. Also plan for additional flexible time so that you can achieve any goals that were not fulfilled. For example, if your goal was to test three children on Monday but two children were sick and you could not test them, you should have another day during the week available on which you can test additional children (e.g., "If I do not reach my goal on Monday, I will cancel my day at the beach on Saturday and test additional children then."). As I noted earlier, research with children demands a special passion and perseverance. You should also have a plan in mind for how best to use your time when children do not make it to a testing session. Will you organize your materials? Will you write? Will you code? Will you call other participants? Always have a backup plan in mind.

Do you have any other tips?

It is easy to get distracted. Before you start doing your research (which can mean anything from recruiting participants to writing a paper), clear your head. While doing your research you cannot be simultaneously worrying about all the other things you need to do—whether it is paying your bills, doing the laundry, or buying your friend a birthday present. Manage your time closely so that, when doing your research, that is *all* that you are doing (i.e., you should not be on Twitter, Facebook, etc., unless and until you are marketing your research). At times when I was working on this guide, I'd make it a special point to occasionally unplug myself from the Internet so that I would not even be tempted to check for emails or the latest news.

 Shut off your cell phone's ringer. Eat and drink enough so that you are not distracted by hunger pangs or thirstiness while recruiting participants or writing your paper. Avoid unnecessary conversations in the hallway.

Of course, you do not want to be antisocial, but you need to immerse yourself thoroughly in the culture of research. Try to schedule your social time carefully, especially if a large project or thesis is due. For instance, you might block out 2–3 hours a week on your calendar for coffee or lunch with colleagues or friends, but the rest of the time you should be hard at work writing or in the laboratory. Try to avoid needless arguments, distractions, and drama; doing so will make you a much more efficient child development researcher.

It sounds easy! Any other tips?

Have you ever planned to go on a trip and cancelled it at the last minute? After doing that, you probably felt suddenly that you had extra time on your hands because you had nothing specific scheduled for the week. Sometimes, to get your research or writing done efficiently, you need to schedule it officially, marking research and writing into your event calendar. Then, when someone asks, "Can we meet Tuesday for coffee?," you look at your calendar and say, "No, sorry, I am booked then. How is Thursday at 4 [i.e., your scheduled social time]?" While all might sound very boring and antisocial, this book, after all, is titled *Doing Developmental Research*, not *How to Be Sociable*.

Try dividing large formidable tasks into smaller, more manageable ones. If your dissertation involves three large studies, try developing a plan to complete the first study before you begin worrying too much about studies two and three. Develop a strategic plan: "By October 10, I will have completed testing 10 babies. By November 1, I will have completed testing 20 babies. By November 15, I will have completed testing 30 babies." Breaking up your goals into smaller segments can help you manage your time better and can make the work ahead seem less daunting.

Summary (check off your achievements)

- Develop a reasonable plan for success. _____
- Always think ahead. _____
- Do your research for the right reasons. _____
- Chose your optimal times and settings for writing. _____
- Develop a workable writing routine. _____
- Set time aside on your calendar specifically for research. _____
- Monitor your goals daily. _____
- Break up large goals into smaller manageable segments. _____
- Set time aside to complete goals you did not achieve the day before. _____

EXERCISES

1. What are your research goals for the week? What are your research goals for today? How will you achieve these goals? (Of course, you can use extra pages from your research notebook.) What will you do if you are unable to achieve those goals? What is your backup plan for alternative goals or activities?

_____

_____

_____

_____

_____

_____

2. Can you think of any guidelines to implement that would better organize your laboratory or team? How might these help new members of your laboratory or the team that you are involved in? List your ideas below, and develop a strategic plan. In this plan, how will you get from point *A* to *B*? What are the mechanisms that you will use?

_____

_____

_____

_____

_____

_____

3. Select a goal. It can be anything from being sure to call your mother, or to write five pages a day, to doing 20 push-ups each morning (see the example below; but select something different from these examples).

I will begin by doing three push-ups each morning before 7 A.M. As a reward, I will have a coffee after I do my pushups. Each day, I will try to increase the number of push-ups by one until I reach 20. I plan to achieve this goal by the end of November (in less than 1 month). If I do not reach this goal, I will not allow myself to buy ice cream for 60 days.

_____

_____

_____

_____

What are your research goals for the day? How will you achieve these goals?

_____

_____

_____

_____

_____

_____

What are your research goals for the week? How will you achieve these goals?

_____

_____

_____

_____

_____

_____

What are your research goals for the month? How will you achieve these goals?

_____

_____

_____

_____

_____

4. Take a look at 10 research laboratories from around the world. (There is space here for three labs. Use your research notebook for additional labs.) Spend 10 minutes apiece investigating how these various laboratories are organized. Everything from the way that participants are recruited to how the lab is organized might give you ideas about how to get your research done more effectively. What did you find? Some examples are listed below.

Golden Meadow Laboratory at the University of Chicago
http://golden-meadow-lab.uchicago.edu
Online schedule of lab meetings and events!
There is a list of prior lab members that even includes their email addresses!
There is a downloadable lab equipment checkout guide!

Infant Development Research Center at Florida International University
http://infantlab.fiu.edu/Infant_Lab.htm
Student award page (great for building the culture of research!).
Related links page, including links to information on child care and parenting.
Conference presentations, with links to posters to download!

Laboratory for Developmental Studies at Harvard University
www.wjh.harvard.edu/~lds/index.html?spelke.html
A wonderful, easy-to-find newsletter about the lab's research.
A great video: "click here to watch a video of a typical infant study."
An easy-to-fill-out online form for recruitment.

Birkbeck Babylab at University College London
www.cbcd.bbk.ac.uk/babylab
A sample of stimuli videos from various studies.
Great use of social media!
Great Facebook link (not to mention a very active Facebook page)!
Nice logo!

Adolescent Stress and Emotion Lab at Arizona State University
https://psychology.clas.asu.edu/doane
Great picture of the team.

Lab Name: _____

Pros: _____

_____

_____

Lab Name: _____

Pros: _____

_____

_____

Lab Name: _____

Pros: _____

_____

_____

5. If you are involved in a laboratory, how do you plan to implement changes in the lab that you consider helpful? What is the timeline for these changes? Who is doing what and when? How might these changes best be achieved?

_____

_____

_____

_____

_____

_____

6. If your lifestyle allows it, deliberately shut down all your access to social media, phone, etc., for 2 hours. What did you do during this time?

_____

_____

_____

_____

_____

_____

_____

7. List in detail what you did for the past 30 minutes.

_____

_____

_____

_____

_____

_____

_____

8. Take 40 uninterrupted minutes to read a peer-reviewed paper or a paper assigned to you. Next, stand alone in a dark, quiet room with your eyes shut for 10 minutes (have someone time you). Answer each of the following questions in a single sentence.

What is the question the paper addressed? _____

_____

_____

_____

_____

Why was this question important? _____

_____

_____

_____

_____

What was new about the findings or the study? _____

_____

_____

_____

_____

Discussion question: How did spending 10 minutes with your eyes closed affect your ability to answer these questions? _____

_____

_____

_____

_____

_____

_____

_____

_____

_____

_____

_____

_____

CONTRACT/TIMELINE EXAMPLE

Date: _August 11, 2011_

Course: _Honors Project_

Semester: _2 of X_

Your Name: _Jane Smith_

Goals as agreed with your mentor/supervisor:

Attend weekly lab meetings.

Recruit and test 10 more 7-month-old infants (providing data that can be
_   used in final study)._

Code (e.g., smiling and gazing) for the 10 infants, and enter the resulting data
_   into SPSS._

Write up the results of the project.

Timeline*:

Recruit 10 infants by October 15.

Test all 10 infants by November 25.

Code infants by December 10.

Write up methods and results by December 20.

Meet with my professor on December 20.

Notes: _Present my progress at the lab meeting on December 6._

Name (supervisor): _____

Signature: _____ Date: _____

Name (supervisor): _____

Signature: _____ Date: _____

*Let your supervisor know if this timeline cannot be met, and immediately determine whether a mutually agreeable alternative timeline can be established.

CONTRACT/TIMELINE

Date: _____

Course: _____

Semester: _____

Your Name: _____

Goals as agreed with your mentor/supervisor:

_____

_____

_____

_____

_____

_____

Timeline*:

_____

_____

_____

_____

_____

Notes: _____

Name (supervisor): _____

Signature: _____ Date: _____

Name (supervisor): _____

Signature: _____ Date: _____

*Let your supervisor know if this timeline cannot be met, and immediately determine whether a mutually agreeable alternative timeline can be established.

LAB SIGN-IN SHEET

Name	Date	Time IN	Time OUT	Accomplishments (be specific)	Comments

CHAPTER 4

Developing Your Ideas and Immersing Yourself in the Culture of Research

Build a network. Get to know your peers and more senior researchers in the field.
—Dr. Stefanie Hoehl, Assistant Professor, Heidelberg University

You may feel like jumping right into your own research project. However, there are some advantages to observing and learning first from others. If there are many research studies going on in the lab that you are working in, then at first perhaps you should simply observe and mainly help out. With the permission of the laboratory director, you might also begin looking at the video records of infants and children who have participated in past studies. Ideally, you should carefully read the research papers that the videos correspond to simultaneously. If your laboratory does not use videotapes, inquire whether other resources exist to help you learn more. Also always strive to learn from people who have been in the laboratory longer than you. Your mentor may have new students starting up in the laboratory as an older group is moving on. One reason for this type of work overlap is that the newest members can learn firsthand from the more seasoned lab members as they rotate out. Learn everything you can from those who precede you. Ask others about their projects, what worked for them, and what they would have done differently. Ask about their time management strategies and how their research experience has helped prepare them for their future career or graduate school.

I feel like I have no research ideas. What should I do?

Once you have figured out the basics of how the lab operates, you should begin thinking about possible research topics. To stimulate and further develop your ideas, it pays to be active in the laboratory, to attend meetings, and to help out on projects even when they are not yours. As a graduate student, I did research on hand–eye coordination in young infants. I would often help the honors students in the lab as they were working on research related to early social expectations. As a result of observing babies in various studies, I was able to develop new questions and new insights about the ways that babies learn about and from the social world. My research focus evolved naturally just by my helping out in the lab. Sometimes, just being interested and curious, can stimulate greater productivity and inspiration in you. If your lab is particularly small, inquire whether you can observe research taking place in other laboratories.

As you develop your research ideas, try to observe and interact with as many infants and children as you can. You might observe them randomly and casually at the toy store, at the zoo, or at restaurants. Watching how children behave in natural contexts will help you to become more familiar with their habits and proclivities, in the end enabling you to become a better researcher.

How can I immerse myself in the culture of research?

To do efficient child development research (or any research, for that matter), you want to invest as much of your energy and resources as possible into, first, developing your research question, then recruiting and testing infants and children, and finally writing up your grant applications and papers. You need to find and then immerse yourself in the culture of research. You might be best advised to "think outside of the box" when looking for inspiration. Look at working places that appear to have a good research culture, and follow their lead. Even if you are not at a major research institute, you can still take small steps to build up your own culture of research. If you are not at a university that fosters or promotes innovation, learn about external programs that do and try to get involved with them. For example, you might take a free online course to get yourself motivated or perhaps watch some online talks from conferences and workshops. I often find myself on Stanford University's "ECorner" website for entrepreneurship learning (*http://ecorner.stanford.edu*) and become motivated by listening to pod-casts and lectures there. Many leading colleges and universities have similar resources available.

> To build a culture of research, open minds and new ideas are essential. If you have an open mind, if you are not bound to hierarchical orders in your lab, you can inspire yourself and inspire the people around you, especially those you are in charge of!
>
> Go to talks and listen attentively, think about it and ask critical questions afterwards. Make an effort to understand other researchers' work. In turn, be prepared to talk about your own interests and ideas. Welcome critical input! This is the input that will help you to go one step ahead. In fact, it might be best to disclose the vulnerabilities of your work. They should be discussed, better sooner than later, because later you will be invested much more and be much less willing to adapt. Don't be overly sensitive if others criticize your work. Take every useful piece of advice and make the most of it, but dismiss messages that will not help you.
>
> If you are already in charge of a small group of researchers, for example, undergraduate students, motivate them as best you can. They are your best help. Organize small meetings, for example a literature group, where you read articles and discuss together. If they are truly interested, you can learn from them.
>
> —Stefanie Peykarjou, MA, Heidelberg University

How to Immerse Yourself in the Culture of Research?

- Sign up for relevant mailing lists.
- Organize a monthly or bimonthly research meeting or brown bag luncheon with researchers and students in your community.
- Update professional posters about upcoming talks, and remove those that are out of date.
- Remove posters at your university that are not parent- or child-friendly.

- Send your recent publications and abstracts to peers as well as scholars you meet at conferences.
- Send a researcher a note to let him or her know you enjoyed reading his or her latest journal article.
- Hold science-in-the-city/-park events.
- Start a monthly newsletter for parents and educators.
- Visit other labs in the vicinity.
- Host a luncheon or breakfast at the laboratory, inviting the public to attend.
- Organize a conference or symposium.
- Volunteer to give a presentation at your next lab meeting.
- Start a Twitter account! Focusing on hashtag (#) entries, look up terms relevant to your research area. You will be amazed at how social media can help foster a "virtual" culture of research and inspire you.
- Hold a "lab organization" party event.
- Start a meet-up group. My laboratory made some fantastic connections with parents and researchers and had fun along the way.
- Join social media sites such as *academia-net.org*, *academia.edu*, or *researchgate.net*, and follow researchers.
- Attend talks at other universities and foundations.
- Hold a meeting to discuss the highlights of a recent conference.
- Participate actively at lab meetings.
- Volunteer to host a guest scientist at a lunch seminar.
- Get to know past and present students in your laboratory.
- Start a research paper club.
- Share a research video or online lecture with colleagues and peers.
- Organize a lab cultural evening or event.
- Develop a newsletter based on your field's latest research findings.
- Did you get a paper accepted? Did your lab mate get into graduate school? Celebrate the success!

I feel like I'm not creative. What should I do?

You will need to have a positive attitude if you want to work with infants and children—or to do *any* research, for that matter. The best researchers typically have creative, open minds and are free-spirited. Whether you are trying to figure out how to get a 1-month-old to look at a computer screen for 30 seconds, a 7-year-old to wait half-a-second before responding to a question, or an active 18-month-old to sit on the floor for 5 minutes, sometimes you need to be very clever and creative as you search out solutions. Solving problems and figuring out the mysteries of human development are what you do as an infant and child development researcher. Because infant and child development happens so rapidly and is influenced by so many factors, there are special challenges that you will face as a researcher. You will need to be persistent and patient as you strive to reach your goals.

On the positive side, doing research can be like riding a bike or playing a competitive sport that you enjoy: that is, once you get the hang of it, it can be fun and at times automatic. I always have a hard time convincing the students in my Intro Research Methods class of this fact, but after a few weeks even the newest researchers admit to finding it fun! As with playing a sport, research can be both competitive *and* fun. It can give you a great sense of achievement and joy to find answers to your questions and to make new discoveries. It can also give you a great sense of accomplishment to complete your thesis or your first publication.

 Be curious. If you want to make it as a researcher or if you want to get the most out of working in a laboratory, stay current on the latest literature, read papers in the field, ask questions, and be prepared to critique the latest trends and developments in the field.

Team sport or solo?

Research is often like playing a sport. If you want to complete your project(s), sometimes you have to tell yourself (just as when competing athletically), "No pain, no gain!" In much the same way that a professional soccer player might end up with torn ligaments and aching joints after an intense match, professional researchers/students may end up with a mild case of the yawns or black circles under their eyes from too much reading! Do you prefer to play soccer (a team sport) or tennis (which is all about you)? There are advantages and disadvantages to doing research as part of a team versus alone. Given the many complicated aspects of conducting research on infants and children, it is usually most common to conduct this type of research as part of a team. A quick survey of the papers published shows that the majority are done by teams. Before I read a research paper, I am always interested in looking at the whole team and the affiliations of its members. The researchers' affiliations are most often listed at the top of the paper near their names. If you are new to research, start paying close attention to such details. You may be surprised to learn that particular laboratories and international teams of senior and junior researchers repeatedly work together.

You don't need to be an expert, but at least know who the experts *are*.

Whenever you are using methods or approaches that are new to you, do not hesitate to speak with experts—and, ideally, get their advice or collaborate with them before diving in. You don't have to know everything—you just need to know who knows what you don't know and develop strong cooperative links and partnerships with them. Doing so can lead to enhanced research speed and effectiveness through wonderful and fruitful collaborations.

How should I form my research team?

Even if you are working on your own honors thesis, you may be a team leader responsible for overseeing many others. Whether engaged in recruitment or testing, you may be working with other students and assistants. No matter what your current research level is, always think about how to manage your team to maximize your research effectiveness.

Put together your research team in much the same way you would go about putting together a good soccer team (or perhaps organizing a good party, if you are not a sports fan). In soccer, you have your goalie, the defenders, the midfielders, and the attack men (forwards, or strikers). Each player has various strengths and weaknesses, some being more versatile than others (e.g., occasionally a goalie is also a great midfielder). In the research world, sometimes the person who is best at coding data is also highly talented at writing up the first draft of the paper. Do you want a stronger product? Carefully developing your team and honing their skills can enable you to develop a better product. Sometimes building a team of people who think differently can aid in developing a superior final product. Perhaps you know someone writing a thesis in the art department or the computer science department or the music department. You never know when people of diverse but unrelated talents might end up contributing usefully to your final product.

Bounce ideas off each other!

It is great to have scheduled lunches with colleagues as settings for discussing thorny questions and research problems that you are working on. Most studies and grants that ever came out of my lab were developed over great times spent with colleagues who were also friends.

 Invite peers from a variety of academic disciplines to your lab meetings. Think outside the box, and try to take an interdisciplinary approach as you learn from peers and colleagues in related fields. This approach can also be very helpful when you are seeking research funding for innovative projects.

Summary (check off your achievements)

- Get to know your peers. _____

- Always be fully engaged at lab meetings. _____

- Keep up with the most relevant literature. _____

- Consider employing an interdisciplinary approach. _____

- Maximize your team's potential by considering individual members' strengths and weaknesses. _____

- Follow relevant research and researchers through the social media. _____

- Celebrate any success you encounter. _____

1. Find two to three research papers, and illustrate the setup of the study. Ask a lab mate or classmate to do the same with the same study. Do your images look similar? Why or why not? (If the setups used in the research studies are clearly spelled out, your images will likely be similar to each other's.)

Paper 1 Title: _____

Image:

Paper 2 Title: _____

Image:

Paper 3 Title: _____

Image:

---

2. The Internet (through such websites as YouTube, Pinterest, etc.) provides you the opportunity to get a "feel" for research. Many journals and laboratories also have videos available online. Here's a link from one of my classes: _http://pinterest.com/triciastriano/professor-tricia-striano_. Watching videos from other laboratories is one way to become familiar with various research paradigms and techniques. You may also get ideas about everything from how to position or hold a baby during a study to what sorts of stimuli other labs use in research studies. Find 10 videos. List the sources here. Share your observations with the class or laboratory, or perhaps even add them to your own social media site. Did watching these videos inspire any research questions? What are they?

_____

_____

_____

_____

_____

_____

_____

_____

3. Describe the scenes/setups shown in Figures 4.1 and 4.2. Copy your descriptions and give them to someone without showing him or her the images. Can he or she draw the setups based on your descriptions? This exercise will help you better describe the setups in your own research paper. Repeat this procedure with your own images.

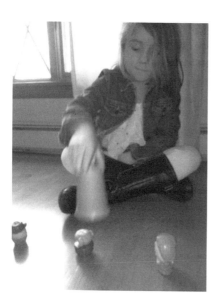 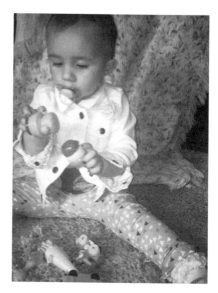

FIGURE 4.1   **FIGURE 4.2**

_____

_____

_____

_____

_____

_____

_____

_____

_____

4. Visit a local park and observe the children's interaction at the playground. What differences did you observe in the boys' behavior versus the girls'? Which behaviors did you compare and why? Next, visit the park with a classmate or friend. Independently define "smile," and then select two children and count the number of times they smile. Were your numbers the same or different? Now, agree upon a definition of "smile" with the same classmate or friend. Select a different child, and then compare your answers. You might also find videos online and repeat this exercise.

_____

_____

_____

_____

_____

_____

_____

_____

_____

_____

_____

_____

_____

_____

_____

_____

_____

Define "smile:" _____

_____

_____

_____

Define "smile" with your lab mate or class partner. Is this person the same or different from above? _____

_____

_____

_____

5. Imagine that you are directing a new research study. What is the study? Plan what supplies you will need for your research.

      Binder dedicated to pertinent research papers
      Computer programs: Photoshop? PowerPoint?

_____

_____

_____

_____

_____

_____

_____

_____

_____

6. List your ideas and strategies for immersing yourself in the culture of research.

_____

_____

_____

_____

_____

_____

_____

_____

_____

_____

_____

_____

_____

_____

_____

7. Find a problem and develop a solution. For example:

Problem: I called the lab and nobody answered.
Solution: Purchase and set up an answering machine.

Problem: The elevator does not function.
Solution: Make signs pointing to the stairs.

Problem: _____

Solution: _____

Problem: _____

Solution: _____

Problem: _____

Solution: _____

Problem: _____

Solution: _____

Problem: _____

Solution: _____

Problem: _____

Solution: _____

8. Make a list of relevant research-related talks and events in your community occurring this month. Do not forget to consider museums, theaters, clubs, and any other relevant venues.

CHAPTER 5

Developing Your Research Question and Proposal

Define your question.

You should be able to ask your research question in a precise way. Think about the meaning of your question. Does it imply that you will be running a correlation or an analysis of variance (ANOVA)? Keep that in mind as you are planning and developing your research question. In most cases, your research question is directly related to previously published research; so, one of the best ways to get started is to read as much related literature in the field as you can. You will notice that many research papers end with a discussion of future directions and open questions. This is often a good place to start as you seek to define your question. Once you have settled on a general subject of interest, begin doing additional research by conducting a literature search. If your question is too broad—for example, "How do children communicate?"—you will naturally be overwhelmed by the number of results returned. You might begin then focusing your literature search on a particular age or situation: "How do young infants communicate through facial expressions?" or "How do infants communicate with siblings?" In the process of reading and learning from the related academic literature, you will discover that there are gaps or open questions to address. As you read the literature, learn from the end-of-chapter exercises, in this book, and also write your ideas in your notebook. You will always be addressing:

1. What is the **question**?
2. Why is it **important**?
3. What is **new** about the study (what does it add to the literature that other studies did not)?

By the time you have read 10–50 papers on a topic, you will have a much better sense about where the important gaps in knowledge really are and hopefully be inspired to address one or two of these gaps. The knowledge that you gain from reading these papers will also help you to write your own papers. You will likely notice a wide range of writing styles and approaches along the way.

> *Plan ahead. Know what statistical tests you are going to use before starting data acquisition, and design your study accordingly. Calculate the resources that will be required realistically (subjects, lab space, time, etc.).*
> —Dr. Stefanie Hoehl, Assistant Professor, Heidelberg University

I'm overwhelmed. What information should my research proposal include?

You should not worry about how many words your proposal should be until you have identified your question. Whether you need to write a 100-page thesis with a complete literature review or simply a manuscript for a journal article, if one were to visualize your thesis introduction or your thesis proposal it would look like a kitchen funnel. Present overarching themes before the specifics and the more generic questions before the more specific ones. Your papers and proposal should focus on three main points (as noted above), namely:

1. What is the question?
2. Why is it important?
3. What's new?

It is easy to write papers, talk scripts, and proposals if you stick to this approach. Do you have a question about which behaviors to code in children? Do you want to know whether your study should use a cross-sectional or, rather, a longitudinal design? The answer is always the same: ask yourself, **"What's the question?"**

One of the best ways to keep track of your research question is to write it down in your research notebook. As you are reading research papers, you should be able to identify what major question was addressed in each one. Identifying the question in one sentence and what was found (i.e., what was new) can help you to develop background knowledge for your own research or review papers.

To begin your thesis proposal, you will want to know . . . ?

"Is my final product to be a journal article?" If so, look at some other examples of journal articles. Ask your thesis advisor or peers in your lab, "Will my thesis be bound and placed in the university library?" One of the best things about writing your thesis proposal carefully is that, if you do a thorough job from the start, you are then one giant step closer to completing your final project. In many cases, in a sense all you have to do is collect your data and fill in the blanks of your proposal. Whether it is a dissertation or an honors or independent study project, before you begin writing your proposal, try to estimate how many pages your final product will be. The longer your final product, the longer your proposal should most likely be. That said, length alone does not necessarily translate into a better product or imply more time productively spent or value created. When students ask "How long should my thesis be?," my reply typically is "It's not about quantity, but *quality*." Generally, a final thesis ranges anywhere from 15 to 100 pages (often chiefly a function of the program requirements and each student's decision), and the final product is ideally submitted in the form of a full-length journal article, which may then be reduced to a brief report.

If you are not sure where to begin, you might best start with a brief introduction of some two to four double-spaced pages (that address the three points of "What's the question, why is it important, and what is new about this study?"); a complete methods section that includes who the anticipated participants will be as well as how they will be recruited; a coding and results section (about three to four pages) that includes anticipated statistics and results, and a full list of references that you plan to include in the final paper and perhaps the full proposal (about one page). One way to start is to show your mentor references of up to 50 research papers that you are considering reading. From these, your mentor might help you select or rank the most relevant ones to read. Check with your mentor for specific guidelines about the required length and format of any anticipated final product. There often is considerable variability across laboratories and universities. Remember when you are writing your methods section that someday someone may seek to replicate your study. Therefore, be very specific when describing the setup and procedures so that even a newly arrived space alien could readily replicate it! Describe your methods as though you were directing a film or a Broadway show (i.e., describe, as it were, the stage and backdrop, what the actors say and do, and where they are in relation to the stage and one another). If someone on stage picks up a vase, give the reader a sense of the vase—is it 5 inches wide or 5 *feet* wide? Is it full of water (if so, say so)? In other words, if a child is looking at a stimulus on a screen, is the screen 12 inches in diameter or 12 feet? Are the lights in the room on or off? Use clear, direct, and ideally short sentences (especially if you are a nonnative speaker). Once again, remember that someone may want to replicate your study some 5 or even 50 years from now. Once your mentor has approved your proposal, you will immediately begin to fill in the introduction with additional details as you begin with collecting data. The skeleton of your final product is now complete. Continue to work to flesh it out each week, and include any progress made in your time management plan. How much are you planning to write each week? Based on this goal, when will your writing be complete (with the exception of filling in the final results and then discussing them).

There are so many research papers to choose from. How can I tell if I am reading a chapter from a larger volume or a peer-reviewed paper?

A peer-reviewed or empirical paper differs in several respects from a secondary source, typically a book chapter. There are often several cues whenever you are reading a peer-reviewed journal paper. You will likely notice a journal title at the top of the paper. To provide an illustration, I selected a research paper titled, "'Did You Call Me?': 5-Month-Old

Infants' Own Name Guides Their Attention," which can be downloaded from the open-access journal *PLoS ONE* at *www.plosone.org/plosone/ article?id=10.1371/journal.pone.0014208.*

The first page of the research paper (see Figure 5.1) gives us several clues. On the top-left corner, you see a little lock symbol and the words "open access." This means that a subscription to the journal is not required to read or access the paper. As you search for research papers using databases available at your local or university library, you will find that some papers require a subscription. If your library does not have a subscription to the journal, you should inquire with your reference librarian about interlibrary loan options. In most cases, it is possible to find a way to access a research paper without incurring any changes. Next to "open access," you may see the words "peer-reviewed" on the online version of the paper. Notations in the online version of this journal made it rather easy for us to see that the paper is peer-reviewed. If it is not obvious, visit the website of the journal. Chapters in books and review papers in journals are also often peer-reviewed. You can normally find out if a journal is peer-reviewed by visiting the journal's website. The listing of a journal editor and editorial board is often a very good indication that papers in that source are peer-reviewed.

The journal information is generally noted on the top and bottom of the research papers. For example, the paper above is published in the journal *PLoS ONE*, as you can see in the top-right header. Under the terms "open access" and "peer-reviewed" we read, "research article." It is common for research articles to indicate this on the report or in the journal's table of contents. Occasionally you will also see the term "report" or "brief report." A brief report is normally a shorter research article. If we further examine the first page of the paper, we can see listed the authors' names and affiliations. In the online version, you can also find out contact information for the authors if you click on the email symbol next to their names. You may wish to contact the authors if you have questions about the paper, or perhaps if you want to expand upon the study and have questions about the procedures. If a paper is coauthored, the "corresponding author" is generally the person who interacts directly with the journal editor and answers readers' queries.

Under the authors' names, you can see that the paper was published on December 3, 2010. The DOI of the paper, or "digital object identifier," is a permanent number used to identify digital information, such as an electronic document. The DOI for this particular paper is

OPEN ⓐ ACCESS Freely available online

"Did You Call Me?" 5-Month-Old Infants Own Name Guides Their Attention

Eugenio Parise[1,2]*, Angela D. Friederici[1], Tricia Striano[1,3]*

1 Max Planck Institute for Human Cognitive and Brain Sciences, Leipzig, Germany, 2 Cognitive Development Center, Central European University, Budapest, Hungary, 3 Department of Psychology, Hunter College, New York, New York, United States of America

Abstract

An infant's own name is a unique social cue. Infants are sensitive to their own name by 4 months of age, but whether they use their names as a social cue is unknown. Electroencephalogram (EEG) was measured as infants heard their own name or stranger's names and while looking at novel objects. Event related brain potentials (ERPs) in response to names revealed that infants differentiate their own name from stranger names from the first phoneme. The amplitude of the ERPs to objects indicated that infants attended more to objects after hearing their own names compared to another name. Thus, by 5 months of age infants not only detect their name, but also use it as a social cue to guide their attention to events and objects in the world.

Citation: Parise E, Friederici AD, Striano T (2010) "Did You Call Me?" 5-Month-Old Infants Own Name Guides Their Attention. PLoS ONE 5(12): e14208. doi:10.1371/journal.pone.0014208

Editor: Antoni Rodriguez-Fornells, University of Barcelona, Spain

Received February 17, 2010; Accepted November 5, 2010; Published December 3, 2010

Funding: This research was supported by the Sofja Kovalevskaja Award granted by the Alexander von Humboldt Foundation, donated by the German Federal Ministry of Education and Research, to T. Striano (http://www.humboldt-foundation.de/web/start.html). In addition, E. Parise was funded by a Humboldt Research Fellowship and by a grant from Calabria Region, Italy (http://www.regione.calabria.it/ricerca). The funders had no role in study design, data collection and analysis, decision to publish, or preparation of the manuscript.

Competing Interests: The authors have declared that no competing interests exist.

* E-mail: eugenioparise@tiscali.it (EP); tstriano@hunter.cuny.edu (TS)

Introduction

Infants are highly sensitive to the communicative social cues that others offer [1,2]. Most infants experience social signals such as eye contact and smiling. Direct eye contact modulates infants' cognitive processes such as face [3,4] and emotion [5,6], and object processing [7,8]. For a review see [9].

Infants use others' social cues to guide their attention to the world. They show enhanced attention to objects that have been cued by joint attention cues such as eye contact and positive facial expressions [2]. In event related potential (ERP) studies, infants show an enhanced Negative central (Nc) component to objects cued by joint attention [7,8]. The Nc is a well-known component related to infant recognition memory [10,11] and enhanced cognitive attentional processing [12,13]. ERP waveforms following the Nc may be involved in maintaining the information over a period of time. They are related to novelty detection [11,14] and to attention [12,15]. For a review see [16]. Infants increase attention when objects are cued by eye contact or joint attention [5,17,18]. However, the question remains whether other social signals are detected and used by young infants when processing the world.

Communicative cues like eye gaze are equal for all infants. But there is one communicative cue that is unique to each individual infant: the infant's own name. Infants' sensitivity to their own first name has only been moderately investigated. Infants listen longer to their own names compared to other names by 4.5 months of age, as demonstrated by the head-turning technique [19]. Infants also respond differently to a close approximation of their own names. If a name differing only in the first phoneme from the infant's own name is heard, infants show no listening preference

[20]. Moreover, 6- but not 4.5-month-olds preferentially respond to the word "baby" but do not show this effect for the word "mommy". This suggests that infants listen preferentially to words typically directed to themselves, such as their own names and "baby".

Research has focused on the role of the infant's own name in early language development. It has been hypothesized that infants use their own name to identify the next word in the speech stream. Available data are inconclusive. Mandel-Emer and Jusczyk [20] failed to provide data supporting this claim. However, they found that 6-month-olds preferentially listen to sentences containing their own name, compared to sentences containing strangers' names. Bortfeld, Morgan, Golinkoff and Rathbun [21] found that 6-month-olds prefer words that, in previously familiarized sentences, were preceded by their own name. This ability was present for the word "mommy" as well, but not for the word "Tommy", suggesting that infants use the first phoneme to differentiate between the two words. Differences in experimental procedures may explain these contradictory results.

A stable and detailed representation of one's own name plays a role in language acquisition, but might also be important in social interaction. Neuroscience research in adults suggests that the own name is special. Using a passive listening oddball paradigm, Folmer and Yingling [22] found an auditory P3 component only in response to the subject's own name compared to other first names. When uttered by a familiar voice, an own name elicits more robust ERP responses of involuntary attention switching (a P3, but also a Mismatch negativity (MMN), respectively related to target recognition and automatic pre-attentive detection to changes in repetitive stimulation) and a large late slow wave at parietal sites [23] (this slow wave is taken to reflect brain activity

FIGURE 5.1

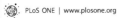

81

10.1371/journal.pone.0014208/journal.pone.0014208. If you enter this DOI into a search engine, the paper appears immediately online. Also on the first page of the paper, you may find other relevant details. Occasionally these details will appear in other sections of the paper, depending on the particular journal. In Figure 5.1, we see the citation of the paper, which includes the authors, year of publication, title, journal, issue, and volume number as well as page numbers and the DOI. Also listed is the editor of the paper.

Looking at the "received," "accepted," and "published" notations can tell us how long it took for the paper to go to press. In many cases, there is also information on when a subsequent revision of the paper was returned to the journal. Here you can see that the paper was received by the journal on February 17, 2010, and accepted for publication on November 5, 2010. Most likely, some minor revisions were required given that nearly 9 months elapsed before the paper was accepted for publication. This may sound like a long time, but it is rather typical (something to keep in mind when you are developing your time management plan). We can see that the paper was published on December 3, which is about 1 month after the manuscript was accepted by the journal. There is a great deal of variability in terms of the time it takes for a paper to be printed or published after it is accepted. With the advent of online journals, these delays have generally been reduced. Sometimes it can take up to a year to see an accepted paper in final print in a journal. Next, we see copyright information from the journal. In this case, copyright remains with the author (i.e., Parise et al.) under the terms of a Creative Common Attribution License. This type of license permits "unrestricted use, distribution, and reproduction in any medium, provided the original author and source are credited." In other words, anyone may use or reprint this work as long as the proper citation is given to the authors of the paper and the journal.

 Taking a look at a variety of research papers and journals and getting a sense of the time it took from original date of submission of a research paper to its date of publication may help you in deciding where to submit your own research papers.

The creative commons copyright is becoming more typical, especially with online open access journals; however, you will still often see that restricted journals limit copyright. Often the journal will state something like "Reproduction in any form, including the Internet, is prohibited without prior permission from the journal." Sometimes, when a paper is published, the authors sign a clause that specifies a transfer of copyright to the journal in which the paper is being published. In this case, the authors need to contact the journal if they wish to republish some or all of their own work. Sometimes this happens if an author is writing a book or chapter based in part on their earlier published work. Perhaps they would like to include some text, figures, or images for which they previously transferred the copyright. In this case, they would have to contact the journal or copyright owner, who would then decide whether to grant permission and normally inform them in writing.

The next section typically tells us about the funding sources for the research. Getting research done often costs a great deal. Funds are normally needed for equipment, recruiting participants, and financing the researchers' labor. Private grants from foundations and public grants from such sources as the National Institutes of Health or the National Science Foundation (NSF) are key contributors to funding research. These sources are acknowledged in a section of the research paper that is often overlooked. However, this section can yield important information that can prove valuable when you are searching for funding for your own research projects. In the case of the article cited in Figure 5.1, two grants funded the project. This section also details to whom the grants were awarded. Most granting agencies require that this information be included in published research papers. Lastly, there is a statement on competing interests in which the authors specify whether they are aware of any conflicts or competing interests. For instance, if they consulted for a drug company and then researched the effects of a drug developed by the same company, they would need to acknowledge that in this section.

Peer-reviewed articles are most often published in journals. These are considered primary sources because they present original research and writing. Secondary sources such as news articles and books often describe and discuss primary sources. Sometimes it can be difficult to decide which articles to begin reading and citing in your proposal. As you become more experienced in the field, this will become easier, of course. **One strategy is to make a reference list of 10–50 possible articles and ask your mentor to help you to decide where to begin.** Be sure first to ask your mentor if these should be exclusively primary and peer-reviewed sources.

In the developmental sciences, empirical papers reporting new data usually include separate introduction, methods, results, and reference sections.

How can I tell if a paper is worth reading?

There can be many ways to select the specific journal articles to read. It is often instructive to visit the various journal websites. Many journals now offer numerous open-access papers that impart the general flavor of the journal. If you are totally new to the field, you should probably consult with your mentor about which journals to consider. When you find a great paper, follow up on it by reading some of the references that were cited in it. You might also try looking through a textbook that is used in one of your developmental science classes. Generally, textbooks and secondary sources are full of relevant primary citations and topics. A journal's Eigenfactor score and its typical impact factor may also provide some clues about the potential value of its articles to you. The Eigenfactor score relates to how many people read a particular journal and thus how important that journal may be in its field. It is based on the total number of citations its articles receive over a certain period of time. Larger and wider-based journals such as *Nature* or *Science* therefore have higher Eigenfactor scores, as these are read and cited more frequently. Impact factors tell us how many citations a journal's articles typically received following publication during the ensuing 2 years. Both the Eigenfactor score and impact factor may give you clues about how important a paper may be. If you are trying to decide which 10 papers to begin reading and you have a list of 200, you might want to start with the highest-impact journals and papers by comparing their Eigenfactor scores and impact factors. You might also bring a list of papers to an upcoming lab meeting and ask your peers and mentor which papers are best to start with. Your mentor may have published 200 research papers, but he or she probably has 10 or 20 favorite papers for you to begin reading. In many cases, the papers that researchers consider their top papers or best work do not necessarily correspond with their highest-impact papers. When in doubt, ask which papers you should begin reading, but begin with a solid list. Optimize the use of your time by reading the most relevant and critical sources for your research first.

Research is often a collaborative—even international—endeavor. When you read a journal article, be sure to take a close look at who the authors are, along with their affiliations. This is one way to get more familiar with the key people in the field and to better understand how collaborations and partnerships are developed. Doing so consistently can help supply you with useful ideas about where to go to graduate school or do your postgraduate work.

I'm having a hard time finding relevant references. What should I do?

First, try thinking of alternative relevant search terms. Which search terms did you use? List the specific search words in your log. You may also find relevant search terms in the following:

Electronic Databases

Google Scholar

http://scholar.google.com

ERIC—Education Resources Information Center

www.eric.ed.gov

PubMed

www.ncbi.nlm.nih.gov/sites/entrez

PsycInfo

www.apa.org/psycinfo

PsycArticles

www.apa.org/psycarticles

Psych Web

www.psywww.com

ScienceDirect Web Edition

www.sciencedirect.com

Look at references in the papers that you did find. Think outside the box!

Lost? Confused? Stressed? Writers' block? Never forget the question.

If you ever get stuck and do not know what to write, it is because you have lost sight of the *question*. Always bring your writing back to the question. Keep repeating the question throughout the paper, and then always answer it the same way.

Together with the guidelines given to you, these tips should help you to write a clear and manageable proposal. In addition to the rationale and background for your project (the page count and other details will largely depend on the specific project), you will want to include your intended methods for data collection, planned analyses, planned graphs and tables, recruitment strategies, a timeline, and a reference section. You will end up filling in the blanks as you conduct your research.

What method should I use?

The one that answers your question in the most direct and simple way. Be sure to describe the specific data that you expect to compile in your proposal. You may wish to enter some sample data and compute the relevant statistics on these data before your write this preview section.

What statistics should I compile?

Compile only the relevant statistics needed to address and answer your question. Other questions must await their own answers in the future.

 Your mentors and committee are part of your team. They most likely have lots of experience and want you to succeed. Work with them to develop a stronger study and strategy.

Here are some tips from a successful honors student:

1. *Even if you don't know what your exact topic will be, start gathering research material as early as possible on the general idea of what you want to write about!*

2. *When you start writing, just write out all of your ideas and thoughts. The very first draft does not need to resemble the final research paper.*

3. *Set writing deadlines for yourself (e.g., three pages a week).*

4. *Update your reference list immediately every time you add or remove a source from your thesis.*

5. *Take mental breaks! Go a few days without even looking at your thesis, and then go back to it with a fresh mindset.*

> —Tala Ginsberg, honors graduate of Skidmore College, PhD candidate in speech pathology, New York University.

Summary (check off your achievements)

- Be able to address: "What's your question, why is it important, and what is new about your study?" _____

- Be able to identify the question that is being addressed in each research paper you read. _____

- Look up several journal Eigenfactor scores and impact factors. ___

- Pay attention to authors' affiliations. _____

- Look at each journal's scope (i.e., stated mission and aims). _____

- Learn about journal submission guidelines. _____

- Look at the grant funding associated with a publication of interest to you (often found in the acknowledgment section of the research paper). _____

- Organize a mock study based on your question. _____

- Outline the "skeleton" of your thesis. _____

EXERCISES

1. Consider your research question.

What's the big question that you are addressing? This is an overarching general question that will drive your research and the decisions that you make along the way.

My big question is: _____

_____

_____

_____

What's the specific question that you are addressing?

Write your specific research question on the lines below. (Note that I have not left too much room for your answer. This is because your question should be written in a concise way!)

My specific question is: _____

_____

_____

_____

What literature did you read to inspire this question? Here, cite 10–20 articles in APA format, and summarize each article. (There is space here for 10 articles. Use your research lab log if you need more space for additional articles.)

_____

_____

_____

_____

_____

_____

_____

_____

_____

_____

_____

_____

_____

_____

_____

2. **Draft your research or project team.** Who does what? What is your strategy to achieve your goals? How are the members linked? Think sports team!

Draw a graphical representation of your team and their relationship below.

3. Find six research journals. What is the scope of each journal (as defined in its website and the journal's pages)? _____

_____

_____

_____

_____

_____

_____

List links to journals here.

_____

_____

_____

_____

_____

_____

Copy one journal's statement of its "scope" here.

_____

_____

_____

_____

_____

Imagine that you are submitting a research paper to the journal. What is the title of your paper as a function of each journal's scope, as defined above? Provide six titles for the same research paper. Do these titles reflect the question? Why is the question important, and what is new in your study?

_____

_____

_____

_____

_____

_____

_____

_____

4. Read the submission guidelines of three journals. Which journal(s) would you select for your paper?

1. _____

2. _____

3. _____

Write an abstract for a possible research study. How does the abstract change as a function of each journal's scope and submission guidelines?

_____

_____

_____

_____

_____

_____

_____

_____

_____

_____

CHAPTER 6

Recruitment and Access

Pound the pavement.
—Dr. Megan Swanson, Postdoctoral Scientist, Hunter College

Before you even begin your study, you want to be sure that you will have a sufficient number of available participants to test. This chapter focuses in particular on recruiting infants and children, since special demands are often associated with the recruitment of such special populations. However, whoever your research subjects are, many of the same principles will apply. As you begin writing your study proposal, you should also be thinking seriously about how and where you intend to recruit your infants and children. Recruiting participants is by no means an automatic process. In most cases, in fact, it is the *most difficult* part of conducting research with infants and children. In Chapter 3, we discussed the importance of considering your time constraints as you begin to think about recruiting participants. Unless you are at a university or a research center with a preexisting database of potential recruits, you will have to work very hard to build meaningful relationships. If you are working with newborns, this means getting to know nurses and doctors. If you are working in a school system, you will want to get to know teachers and principals. During your first weeks of using the lab, roughly 5 hours of relationship building may be needed to yield one test of a baby or child in the laboratory. Over time, your relationships and research potential may grow exponentially. But building relationships is not just about writing a post on Facebook or sending a letter to a preschool. It is important to get into the community and really familiarize yourself with the people. Schools, hospitals, and community agencies often want to know how you might add value to *their* programs. For instance, perhaps you might offer to hold an informational session for parents at the school and/or assist the school in offering a special event. Perhaps teachers would like you to come in once a week and read a book to the class or to teach a lesson related to your research. You must always consider, first and foremost, the needs of the parents, children, educators, and community organizers you meet and seek to recruit. Parents are often reluctant to have their children participate in research. This is especially true if you are unable to convey the seriousness and significance of the question you are posing in a clear and concise way. You need to be able to communicate the minimal risks and considerable benefits for the parents and children involved. For instance, what knowledge or experience will parents gain by having their child participate in your research? How might their child benefit concretely? Can you offer a 30-minute class for parents about the subject you are studying? Doing so might give them the opportunity to learn useful information and also to meet other parents. Perhaps the children will appreciate receiving a small educational toy and simultaneously find the experience entertaining and fun. You should also provide ample time to answer any questions that parents may have. You might also want to develop a short video you could show parents or caregivers that addresses what happens when they visit the laboratory or shows how we study children. Ideally, you want to be able to convey some tangible, real benefits that accrue benefits to parents and caregivers for their child's participation.

Contacting people at the right time of day can also make a big difference. If your research involves children, consider their parents. Consider what their day may be like. Do they have other children at home? Do they work full-time? It may be best to call at 10 in the morning rather than at 8 in the evening. When you make your original contact with parents or caregivers, find out the best way to reach them (email, telephone, or text message) and the best time and day. In many places, nannies or day care providers often care for young children during weekdays, but parents are with them on weekends. In such cases, weekend recruitment might be best reserved to parks.

Similarly, when contacting schools you will find that teachers and school administrators are very busy planning and prepping for the school year at the start of the academic year. If you are planning to begin your research study in September, plan ahead and get into contact with school officials the prior March or April. This leaves you May and June to build mutual relationships, develop your strategy, plan networking events, and get your materials approved through the school. In this way, everything is ready once September rolls around.

What about recruitment tips for children with special needs?

Always remember to consider the needs of your participants. This is all the more true of children with special needs. Being a parent of a child with special needs can be exhausting and frightening. Parents may feel that there is no direct relationship between your research study and the outcome of their child's illness or condition. It is important to be sensitive. Take time to get to know the parents, and take time to understand their concerns and their children. Build a meaningful mutual relationship. Here, I can also offer a personal example. When I became an aunt to premature twins, I immediately wanted to get the newborns into a research study (realizing as I did the potential benefits of music and language on brain development and the research that was then occurring in the neonatal intensive care unit [NICU] at the hospital). I immediately contacted the researcher at the NICU where the babies were born and inquired whether they could possibly participate. Hours later, the researcher ran into the new parents in the hospital elevator as they were on their way to the NICU (he noticed their nametags, so he knew they were my relatives!). The next day my sister-in-law told me something about a research study and the encounter with the doctor/researcher in the elevator. But of course research was the last thing on their minds at the time. After having just seen their 1-pound, 13-ounce, and 2-pound babies for the first time, they were solely concerned about the survival of their babies at that point. Some days later, a research assistant spoke to the parents about the study, and they agreed to participate in the research. So, many factors can influence participation in research. Timing can be extremely important. To increase your chance of success, you need to be very sensitive to the particular situation and to the needs of the parents and caregivers as well as your participants in general. For example, if you are working with college students, it is likely better to contact them at the start of the semester rather than during midterms or finals. Before asking if they are interested in participating in research or in learning more about your study, you should probably first ask if you are contacting them at a good time.

Here are some further tips that I received from a colleague who was working with special populations.

1. Pound the pavement (literally), and make local connections (i.e., visit schools, after-school programs, day care programs that serve children with special needs). Offer to come and give a short informational session on your research. All you need is one principal/director to send out your information on their list serve.

2. Referral is key. I always follow up with families after an assessment session to thank them for participating. I ask them how I can be of further assistance and inform them of next steps in the research project (i.e., follow-up visits, when I will have an assessment report ready). I also stuff a couple of extra flyers and my business card in the envelope containing "compensation" (cash) that I give families at the end of an assessment session.

3. Be visible. Have an up-to-date online presence (website, social media). You want families to feel that you are doing current, state-of-the-art research, and that their participation will result in research that will "make a difference." I think that this point is especially important for families of special-needs kids. They need to either feel like they are going to get something out of the research (a report on standardized assessments of language/cognitive skills, treatment, advocacy training), or that their participation is going to improve the lives of future families. Honestly, 80% of my participants came from 10% of the parents/schools/after-school programs that I contacted. The "hit-rate" of recruitment can be quite low, so recruitment strategies should be a comprehensive, continuous effort. I tell my undergrads that recruitment could be a full-time job, especially at the start of the project!

—Dr. Meghan Swanson, Postdoctoral Scientist, Hunter College

Working with the media to help with recruitment

When you are starting up a new area of research, you might even contact the media and see if they would like you to write a summary of recent research findings or a summary description of your lab. This can be a win-win situation: the media receive professional advice and information on infant and child development, and your lab gets complimentary media that may help to attract new parents to your laboratory. Look for local parenting magazines and resources. Think outside the box.

How does socioeconomic status influence how I recruit infants and children?

A variety of factors may influence how and where you recruit infants and children for your studies. Try to think of where your potential participants spend their time, and try to make connections and build trust with those people you will be working with. For instance, if you think you may like to recruit children or parents from a shelter, you might first try to reach out to the director of the shelter for a preliminary face-to-face meeting to discuss your project. Remember that people have limited time, so if you take this approach be sure to show up on time and act professionally. You might leave some materials about your work and subsequently follow up once the director has had time to think about how your work might fit in. You might try to offer some complimentary talks, books, or lectures about your research. Let potential directors and parents know what they could gain by participating in your research or learning more about it. Offering complimentary lectures or question-and-answer sessions is one way to give back to communities for their help.

I'm working with children and teenagers. Any tips on recruiting?

When working with teens, you need to keep in mind their busy schedules and the power and influence of peer pressure. You might want to reach out to school directors to determine the best way to reach your population. Perhaps you could give a presentation during their lunch or break time. Teens will also want to know how they would benefit from taking part and how their sensitive materials will be protected. Getting to know teachers and community leaders can help you in your efforts to get children and teens involved in your research. Branding can also make a difference. You will want to try to connect with teens by having them relate to you and your work. Perhaps you can offer them incentives such as music or a gift certificate from a store that they like.

How do I market my research for different cultures?

No matter what language is involved, you need a great deal of cultural sensitivity to be a fully effective researcher. Try to make children feel comfortable by having an assistant who shares the same native

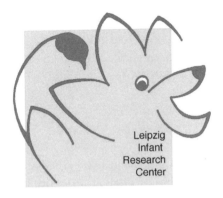

Leipzig
Infant
Research
Center

FIGURE 6.1

language with them. You will also want to have your flyers and consent forms available in their original tongue. You will need to plan ahead if you are not multilingual. Keep the relevant cultural contexts in mind when you are marketing your research.

Culture will also influence your branding. A logo is an important part of branding for your research laboratory and for recruitment in general. Figure 6.1 shows a logo that my research group used at the Max Planck Institute for Human Cognitive and Brain Sciences. It was a playful lion, based on the Leipzig Lions' (soccer team) mascot. You may be part of a larger research center and want to link your logos to other departments, which can be a nice way of expressing solidarity with the wider community of scholars.

Figure 6.2 depicts the logo for the Developmental and Autism Laboratory—"DAL"—of Dr. Roberta Fadda at the University of Cagliari in

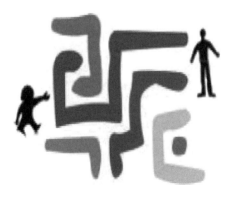

FIGURE 6.2

Sardinia, Italy. I like this logo for several reasons, including the uplifting colors of the maze. The logo reminds us of the puzzle of autism and also the sense of development connecting the baby with the adult. The logo you create should be both meaningful and memorable.

Database: Planning

As you are building your database of participants, keep an Excel chart so that you can closely monitor your progress in recruiting. You might want to present a graph depicting the sample size and its constituent parts at the start of each lab meeting. Are your strategies for recruiting participants working? Are certain ones working better than others? Are there unwanted age gaps among those thus far recruited? How do you plan to solve this problem?

I recruited a child for my study, but the parents did not give permission for me to video record. What should I do?

Communication is the key. Often the manner in which you describe your procedure can make a big difference. Did you explain why you were asking to take the video? Studying infants and children often demands a microanalytic approach. Videos are coded for behaviors in slow motion for smiling, directing one's attention, and various vocalizations. Videotaping is also important because it helps us to establish reliability between coders. Parents and educators are much more likely to agree to having their child recorded if they are permitted to keep a copy for themselves. We have found that parents often enjoy showing the video to their friends and family.

They still said no! Now what?

If you definitely must have a video, go on to recruiting your next participant and do not worry about it.

I had six infants scheduled this weekend, and none showed up! What am I doing wrong?

Did you confirm the appointment at least 24 hours ahead via telephone and also by email? Was your phone message clear and coherent?

How do I schedule and confirm calls?

Speak clearly and confidently: "If you are unable to make your appointment, I'd really appreciate it if you could call me at _____ or send an email to the lab. I look forward to seeing you and [baby/child's name] on [day/date]." Did you give parents an opportunity to change the day of the appointment?

> **TIP:** Do you always ask parents who come into your lab whether they have contacts or friends who might like to visit the lab? Give parents extra promotional materials about your lab to distribute to their friends. Research is about 90% recruitment.

The scripts and flyers that you develop may also influence your success. Some examples from my laboratory are presented on pages 107–109.

Summary (check off your achievements)

- Develop a recruitment strategy. _____
- Always strive to stay. _____
- Ask for referrals. _____
- Hold creative networking events. _____
- Don't miss opportunities. _____
- Keep cultural contexts in mind. _____
- Develop a great brand and logo. _____
- Send out summaries of your research. _____
- Develop relevant scripts. _____

EXERCISES

1. Read "From New Logos to New Coke: 5 Corporate Mistakes" (*http://msn.com/en-us/money/companies/from-new-logos-to-new-coke-5-corporate-mistakes/ar-AAa524k#page-1*) and "15 Worst Corporate Logo Fails" (*www.businessinsider.com/15-worst-corporate-logo-fails-2012-1?op=1*). As you are thinking about the design of your logo, you might also like to watch the film *Helvetics* (*www.helveticafilm.com*). *Helvetica* is a feature-length independent film about typography, graphic design, and global visual culture. It looks at the proliferation of one typeface (which celebrated its 50th birthday in 2007) as part of a larger conversation about the way type affects our lives. The film is an exploration of urban spaces in major cities and the type that inhabits them, and a fluid discussion with renowned designers about their work, the creative process, and the choices and aesthetics behind their use of type (*www.helveticafilm.com/about.html*).

Another relevant film is *Art & Copy* (available on DVD). "ART & COPY is a powerful new film about advertising and inspiration. Directed by Doug Pray (SURFWISE, SCRATCH, HYPE!), it reveals the work and wisdom of some of the most influential advertising creatives of our time—people who've profoundly impacted our culture, yet are virtually unknown outside their industry. Exploding forth from advertising's 'creative revolution' of the 1960s, these artists and writers all brought a surprisingly rebellious spirit to their work in a business more often associated with mediocrity or manipulation: George Lois, Mary Wells, Dan Wieden, Lee Clow, Hal Riney, and others featured in ART & COPY were responsible for 'Just Do It,' 'I Love NY,' 'Where's the Beef?,' 'Got Milk,' 'Think Different,' and brilliant campaigns for everything from cars to presidents. They managed to grab the attention of millions and truly move them. Visually interwoven with their stories, TV satellites are launched, billboards are erected, and the social and cultural impact of their ads are brought to light in this dynamic exploration of art, commerce, and human emotion" (*www.artandcopyfilm.com/synopsis*).

For more on graphic design tips that may help you with recruiting for your study, read *100 Ideas that Changed Graphic Design*, by Steven Heller and Véronique Vienne (published in 2012 by Laurence King Publishing Ltd.).

You have just started your own laboratory that studies cognitive development among 3- to 7-year-olds. Design your logo here.

You have just started your own laboratory that studies stress among college-age students taking research methods classes. Design your logo here.

Show your logo to five people. What are their comments?

_____

_____

_____

_____

_____

_____

_____

_____

_____

_____

Can you improve your logo based on their comments? Why or why not? If so, design another one or two on the next page.

_____

_____

_____

_____

_____

2. Develop a 30-second YouTube commercial for a study that you are conducting in your new laboratory.

3. Swimming lessons, movie theaters, face painting, and library book clubs—the possibilities are endless for recruiting. But you need to be a bit creative! Walk or drive around the area where you plan to conduct your research studies.

Can you find at least 20 signs or events or businesses related to infants and children (see examples in Figures 6.3 and 6.4)? What was your strategy for finding these signs? How long did it take you? How did you manage your time? Take photos and paste them here or on a blog (or bring them to your next lab meeting or class).

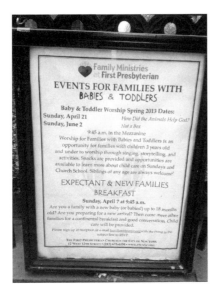

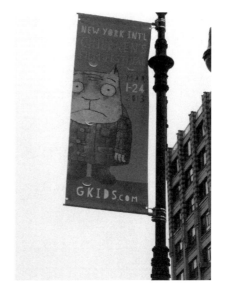

FIGURE 6.3

FIGURE 6.4

4. Pretend you are conducting a study with 5-year-old children. From the parking lot to the laboratory and back, do a run-through of what the parents and children will experience upon arriving at the lab.

Did you see anything inappropriate (include photos if possible)? _____

_____

_____

Would they have any difficulty finding the laboratory? _____

_____

_____

Could anything have gone more smoothly? Why or why not? _____

_____

_____

Develop a script with directions to the laboratory. _____

_____

_____

Could an inexperienced individual find the lab, based on the instructions you provided? _____

_____

How long would it take him or her? _____

_____

Solve all logical problems before you invite participants to the lab. What's your strategy? Write it here. _____

_____

_____

_____

_____

5. Write a telephone script for a research study involving 3-month-old infants. Write a telephone script for a research study involving 15-year-old males.

_____

_____

_____

_____

_____

_____

_____

_____

_____

_____

_____

_____

6. Find three ads for research studies on the web. List the links here.

_____

_____

_____

What are the pros and cons of each? _____

_____

_____

_____

_____

_____

_____

Would you participate in the studies? Why or why not? _____

_____

_____

_____

_____

_____

_____

ADVERTISEMENT

[Your school's letterhead/logo]

Hello, Caregivers!

We are the _____, a new laboratory at [your school's name].
Our aim is to answer many important questions about the early social, cognitive,
and communicative skills of infants and children. Our research helps parents and
caregivers to better understand infant and child development.

Some of the basic questions we now study are:

- Why is eye contact so important?

- How do infants learn?

- Can infants learn from digital media?

- How does language develop?

- We would like to invite you to join our research.

Participation is voluntary.

For additional information, please visit us online at _____.com
or call us at 000-000-0000.

PARENT TELEPHONE SCRIPT

Project Title: Social Monitoring

Hello, my name is _____, and I work in the _____
Laboratory at [school name, college/university]. Your name was selected from
our participant database, which consists of parents who have shown interest in
participating in studies of child development. If it is okay with you, I would like to
invite you and your child _____ [child's name] to participate in a
study in our child development laboratory.

If a positive response is given, the caller will then continue:

Thank you for taking the time to talk with me. I am sure you enjoy being a parent and
that your child brings you a lot of joy! Our Infant and Child Development Research
Laboratory is at [school name] and our lab director, Dr. _____, is
an Assistant/Associate/Professor at [school name's] Department of Psychology. We
study the development of social cognition in infants and children.

I would like to tell you a little bit about the study and will answer any of your
questions. Studies may take place in your child's school or in our Infancy Research
Laboratory at [school name]. We will give your child a small gift such as a T-shirt, box
of crayons, coloring book, or toy as a token of our appreciation. You will receive the
gift even if, once you are at the lab, you decide not to let your child participate in or
complete the study.

Your infant is being asked to participate in a study on early social cues and learning.
We will show your baby several social cues—for example, we may look at an object
and then back to your baby while talking and vocalizing with a positive voice. We will
then show your baby an old object and a new object to determine which one he or
she may prefer. We will video record your infant's behavior. You will be in the room
with your infant for the entire study. The procedure is noninvasive. Participation is
voluntary and unrelated to your infant or child's health. You may choose to end the
testing procedure at any time and need not give a reason for doing so.

If your infant begins fussing during tests, he or she will be given a 2- to 5-minute
break. With your approval, he or she will then resume the testing procedure.
However, if at any point your infant fusses for more than 30 consecutive seconds, the
testing procedure will be ended. Testing will be recorded on video, and therefore we
will ask you to sign a video consent form and a general consent form before testing
begins.

(continued)

We are specialists in the study of typically developing children. Therefore, we are not qualified to diagnose or treat developmental disorders. If you have any concerns about your child's health or development, please discuss them with a pediatrician.

Do you have any additional questions? [Pause to answer questions.]

Are you interested in having your infant participate in our study?

If the answer is "yes," continue with the script below. If the answer is "no," the caller will thank the parent for his or her time and politely say goodbye.

Thank you very much for your willingness to participate. We have testing times available at _____ and _____. What time is convenient for you?

We will send you a copy of our lab's brochure, in which you will find instructions and directions to our lab.

Thank you very much for your time, and please feel free to call or e-mail us with any additional questions.

Goodbye!

CHAPTER 7
Organizing and Planning Your Study

Date is the universal organizer.
—Dr. Philippe Rochat, Professor of Psychology, Emory University

How should I organize my files?

Even before you begin testing your subjects, you want to have a plan for organizing your data. Decide with your research team about the best strategy to organize and date your files if a system is not already in place. If you live in Europe, perhaps you date your files 01–04–2013 instead of April 1, 2013, but if you are collaborating with someone living in the United States, he or she will interpret this date as January 4. It is crucial to use a dating system that will be accurately interpreted by all. Dating files and video records is especially important when you are revising various versions of manuscripts. What's most important is that everyone be *consistent* and know the correct formats and specifications for maintaining an organized and efficient laboratory. "**Date is the universal organizer**" is among the great tips that I learned from my mentor. Always name and date your files (e.g., 30January2014Revised-MSJointAttention3months, as opposed to "revisedMS"). In addition to dating the file name, you will also want to date the text. Remember that someday you may be working on 10 research projects at once, and each project might be in collaboration with colleagues in the United States, New Zealand, and Germany. Prevent disaster and save time by dating and naming any file created and by putting the date (in an agreed-upon format) on each version of any paper you write.

The following are generally good rules to observe:

- Develop a plan for organizing and labeling your files with your research team (you can add this plan to your general lab guidelines).

- Add detailed instructions for dating video records or files. If you record the participant's date of birth on a video record as well as the testing date, you can easily calculate his or her age 5, 10, or 15 years later. Dates and records help you to reconstruct video records accurately, whatever the time frame in question.

- Do not forget to record clearly each participant's gender. Do not automatically assume that a baby dressed in blue is a boy. Be sure your records reflect accurately the child's gender, assigning each one an appropriate ID linked to demographic factors so that you do not have to reinvestigate these later.

- Did something unusual happen during a testing session? Perhaps a parent's cell phone rang or the child got tired and had a snack in the middle of the testing session. Occasionally, as a new researcher, you will be uncertain whether to include a child in a final sample or not. To minimize confusion, keep excellent notes in your lab log, and in difficult cases consult with your mentor, who can help you decide on a case-by-case basis.

This video won't play. What should I do?

One day a student showed me an old videotape that "didn't work," explaining simply that it was labeled "Does Not Work." The problem was that no one knew any of the details or particulars of the labeling. Does the tape make a loud sound when it is being played? Is it completely unplayable? Might it break the player if inserted into the machine? Be sure to provide enough details on the tape itself that, 10 years down the road, anyone who picks up that tape will know exactly what "Does Not Work" means.

One key instruction in efficiently conducting research is to label your files adequately. Give all of your files, especially documents, a clear descriptive title, ideally with an unambiguous date. Do not create files that you then title "manuscript" or "Final version65."

It is easy, as a graduate student, to feel as though you'd love to undertake an ambitious study inspired by questions that are large, complex, and highly significant. You need to be passionate, after all, to be a good researcher, since certain parts of the research process are not much fun—recruiting participants and dealing with reviewers. For example, you need to care deeply about the questions you are asking. However, you also need to appreciate time constraints and therefore to propose studies that are manageable (i.e., practicable). In fact, one of the key aspects of doing successful research is keeping your project under control. That is especially true when testing infants and children, because there is a lot about their behavior that is especially difficult to control—yet, you must stive to control as much as possible. If you need to complete your study within 6 months, just ask yourself, "Is this really possible?" Also, do not assume that, just because similar research has already been published, that it was easy to conduct or complete quickly. Some studies in my lab take only days to complete, whereas others may take years. One cannot predict research studies' timelines accurately, based solely on previously published research. One good idea is to reach out to those familiar with the problems you are likely to encounter and ideally collaborate with them as you learn the ropes. This approach can aid you at several stages of your career.

 Sometimes "less is more." It's amazing what great research can be done with only limited resources. A couple of toys, a pencil, and a stopwatch can get one surprisingly far.

Visiting labs is a great way to become a more capable researcher. Sometimes the places with the least financial resources nonetheless possess the best infrastructures for doing original research. Efficient research often involves accurately assessing your resources and making the most of them.

What design should I use for my study?

To address this question, you simply need to go back to the precise research question that you wrote in your notebook. The question should help you to determine the best design to use. Are you interested in change over time? In that case, perhaps you need a longitudinal design. Are you interested in changes among groups as a function of age? If so, what are the age ranges involved? You should have a strong rationale for all decisions that you make and should avoid including extraneous variables or research subjects (i.e., participants) in your studies.

Measures and designs

I have used exclusively cross-sectional studies, for convenience (it's difficult to get parents to agree to come into the lab just once!) and also to control for practice effects. I would like to do longitudinal research in the future. One design I use frequently is an age-matched control design: infants are the same age, but some other developmental characteristic (locomotor status: crawler vs. walker, walking/crawling experience, etc.) is allowed to vary. This lets us examine effects of the developmental factor independent of age, which allows us to learn more about processes of change. I have used both experimental (measuring infants' responses to an experimentally manipulated variable) and observational (quantifying infants' behaviors when allowed to behave freely) methods, and I find that they complement each other. Experimental studies allow the experimenter more control, but observational studies have ecological validity.
      —Kari Kretch, PhD candidate, Department of Psychology, New York University

Think of everything that can go wrong before you begin, and then methodically consider possible solutions.

As a researcher, you are always looking for a solution or an answer to a problem. One of the best ways to get research done effectively to consider all the problems that might arise and then focus on coming up with solutions.

For example, here are some problems that might arise:

Problem: Baby sliding off parent's lap.

Solution: Demonstrate how the parent should hold the baby. Explain to the parent that sometimes, in the middle of a session, babies can begin to slide and that it is important to keep the infant in place. Sometimes a little extra explaining in advance can make a big difference in outcomes.

Problem: Babies using pacifiers.

Solution: Remove pacifier.

Problem: Siblings in the same room.

Solution: Arrange to have a lab mate babysit any siblings. Check with the parent when scheduling the child whether anyone else will be accompanying them. Check with other lab personnel. Might the sibling be able to participate in a study? Be sure age-appropriate activities are available for the sibling.

Problem: Toys that are not safe for children.

Solution: Check the labels on toys, and never keep toys in the lab that are unsafe.

Problem: Camera battery is running out.

Solution: Make a habit of asking aloud at the start of testing, "Battery okay?" Or develop a verbal or written checklist to go through prior to starting.

Problem: Baby is getting sick.

Solution: Keep cleaning supplies handy.

 One way to figure out what might go wrong is to conduct some pilot lab tests with lab personnel in advance.

I'm conducting a cross-cultural study. Is there anything I should keep in mind?

In another culture, communication may be quite different from your own. Whereas in one culture conflicts are settled directly and in the open, in another culture (sometimes even in only another lab's culture) conflicts may be solved more implicitly. Keep your eyes and ears open and do not take control too early, but get acquainted with the lab's culture.

Not only may the culture of the researchers differ, but also the culture of the participants. For example, in the US, infants and children are talked to in a very excited and exciting way. In other countries, infants may be treated much calmer. Be ready to adapt! It's important for you and for your participants. They should be comfortable, and they need to feel that everything is fine. Only if you can get them to relax will you get usable data, especially if working with infants!

Also, if you are a visiting researcher in a lab, you usually do not have much time to adapt. You have only a limited amount of time, and you wish to do as much as possible—run many subjects, analyze tons of data, finish a study, and write a paper. All this in as little time as possible. Be prepared: This might not work out. Don't be stressed out. Sort your plans according to importance, and do what has to be done. Don't forget to enjoy your time in a different culture—this is a great experience!

—Stefanie Peykarjou, MA, Heidelberg University

More problem prevention

Experimenter stress can influence your results. Try to stay relaxed. Communicate fully and calmly with the parents, and make them feel at home.

"Do you think [baby] is hungry?"

"Does [baby] need to be changed?"

Testing teens? Do they need a break to check their cell phone?

Testing children? Would a snack midway through the test session help them complete the remainder of it?

I'm a new researcher. Do you have any tips as I begin to plan my research?

This is a common question, and to help answer it for you I received some advice from one of my colleagues, Dr. Roberta Fadda, Research Lecturer at the University of Cagliari in Sardinia, Italy. She has had great success in recruiting and working with typically developing children, but also with those with special needs, such as autistic children.

When I was a young researcher, I mainly worked with typically developing children and infants. In my opinion, the key to being successful in the research field was the ability to see the world from the participants' perspective. With this idea in mind, I tried very hard to see the world from the child's perspective. I started by reading a lot of books and papers about child development.

My goal was to learn in detail what a child can think, feel, and understand, in order for me to be able to predict their behavior in a particular experimental setting. However, the translation from knowledge to practice was not as immediate as I wished! Nothing seemed predictable enough. Only after years of experience did I become comfortable in testing infants and children. What changed?

Well, first of all, my priorities changed. When I was a new researcher, my priority was to apply observational protocols in a very rigid way. However, the risk of this strategy was to "lose" the baby. I wanted his/her cooperation and the exact moment of the study to test him/her for a specific ability. I wanted the child to follow my plan. With the experience, having the child involved became my first goal; with practice, I learned that I was ready when the child was ready!

Experience also helped me with flexibility. Testing infants and children, it is likely that some object or stimuli might get lost or accidentally broken. Experience taught me to be flexible. For example, rather than interrupt a testing session I learned to plan ahead and to have some extra materials available.

It is also likely that a child might be tired, upset, and generally not cooperative. In this case, it is important to interrupt the testing and catch the participant when he/she's ready.

To cope with unpredictable situations, I think it's a good idea to run some pilots before the study. Pilots help to familiarize [us] both with the children and with the experimental setting and to develop effective strategies to help with undesirable situations.

Be patient and . . . follow the lead of the baby and . . . give them opportunities to show their abilities when they are focused and motivated. Experience taught me not only to wait but also to be "fast"! Once a baby or child is ready, being rapid in responding to the participants' behavior helps with synchronization in the interaction. This is a good way to keep participants engaged during the testing.

Parents have always been very helpful with advice and suggestions. When I was a new researcher, some parents' opinions appeared to be in conflict with my protocols and plans. Thus, I tended to ignore them. Today I know that was not a good idea. As a young researcher, I didn't realize that parents had the best knowledge of the child and, since they wanted to cooperate with the experiment, they knew the best way to redirect the child and to motivate her/him during the testing.

Here are some of my tips for a young researcher working with a typical baby:

- *Practice with a specific population (especially with infants and children—maybe friends of the family!).*
- *Set strategies to cope with "unexpected" events (e.g., a broken toy).*
- *Be flexible.*
- *Follow the lead of the baby/child (be sensitive and give opportunities for the child to become engaged).*

- *Listen to parents.*
- *Run pilots/practice.*

I plan to work with children with autism. Do you have any special tips?

All these tips are particularly precious when a young researcher works with special populations, like children with autism spectrum disorders. I've been lucky enough to work as a behavioral therapist for children with autism spectrum disorders 3 years before I started to run research on this special population. The advantage to working with them has been the possibility of seeing the world from their perspective, getting used to their special perceptions, beliefs, emotions, and learning to interpret the meaning of their peculiar behaviors and habits.

This knowledge might be gained by volunteering at a school or intervention settings with the population that they are targeting with their research. Volunteering might be a productive way to gain opportunities to meet these children and learn more about them. Following the lead of the parents is a priority with these children, due to their lack of communication and/or social competence. Professionals and teachers might play the same role as the parents if the testing is organized at school or at the hospital. It's good to learn from the professionals. I believe that this practical experience should be combined with a deep knowledge of the distinctive characteristics of these special populations.

—Dr. Roberta Fadda, Research Lecturer, University of Cagliari

If you are testing a special population of children consider having them in for a visit prior to participating. A lab open house can be a great way to familiarize families with the lab and to recruit them for your study. Remember to put yourself mentally in the place of the parent or the baby (i.e., "in their shoes"). From the time the parents arrive at your university or institute, what will they see and how will they feel? Is there a chance they might get lost trying to get there? Did you pre-test your lab directions with 10 sample subjects to ensure they did not encounter any problems in finding the laboratory? Should you plan to meet and greet your prospective participants in the parking lot? Think of everything that might go wrong, and then tackle the problem. The last time my lab tried experimenting with "pretend" participants first arriving for a study (a mother with an infant), we found a sign saying "Both elevators out of order! Take the stairs." Needless to say, we had to improvise a solution on our own.

From preparing labels for tapes and video records to anticipating what condition an infant or child will be in, have all your materials ready ahead of time. Get the laboratory fully in order at least 30 minutes ahead of schedule, to better plan and prepare for the session.

It is important to achieve the right balance in setting the scene for children and infants. If children are to have a warm-up session beforehand, are the toys you give them to play with too exciting? If so, they might not want to participate in your study. Find the right balance through trial and error. Ideally, make your mistakes during pilot sessions rather than during real testing sessions. Practice makes perfect.

One of the best ways to prevent problems with data is to keep very good records and to remain in close contact with your raw data. It is always a good idea to review the raw data regularly. I often ask my students to pull up their data files and then to immediately screen the original videos. I then watch the videos with them and code a few babies myself over the course of the study to ensure scoring reliability and also to be sure that the data files are being compiled and stored correctly.

Summary (check off your achievements)

- Anticipate problems. _____

- Find solutions. _____

- Develop a commonsense organizational system for your data and files. _____

- Date all your files in an unambiguous format. _____

- Date and label all your data records consistently. _____

- Consider cultural differences. _____

- Consider the effects of the immediate environment. _____

- Place yourself in the shoes of the parent. _____

- Place yourself in the shoes of the infant or child. _____

- Ask parents for suggestions, and always remain open-minded in responding to them. _____

EXERCISES

1. What is your plan for titling and dating your files and for naming your research study? If you are not involved in a specific research project, invent one for the purposes of this exercise.

_____

_____

_____

_____

_____

_____

_____

_____

_____

_____

Will someone understand your codes 10 years from now? Why or why not?

_____

_____

_____

_____

_____

_____

_____

_____

_____

2. Read two empirical articles. What could have gone wrong in these studies? Were any precautions taken against adverse consequences that were described in the research paper?

_____

_____

_____

_____

_____

_____

_____

_____

_____

_____

3. Have you ever done research abroad? What are some considerations to keep in mind when conducting a research study abroad?

_____

_____

_____

_____

_____

_____

_____

What special problems apply to a research study focused on various socioeconomic status groups? _____

_____

_____

_____

_____

_____

4. If the setting allows it, literally put yourself in the shoes of a baby. Crawl on your hands and knees for 5 minutes. What do you see and discover?

_____

_____

_____

_____

_____

_____

5. You are designing a study for 10-year-old children. You want children to feel comfortable in the waiting room. What posters do you select to put on the wall and why? Place your Internet links here.

_____

_____

_____

_____

_____

After you test the children, you want them to be in a good mood and listen to some music. What three songs do you select and why? How did you make these selections? What was your rationale? Is it research-based? If so, why or why not?

_____

_____

_____

_____

_____

CHAPTER 8

Strategies for Using Statistics

There is a life behind repeated measurement ANOVA!
—Dr. Daniel Stahl, Senior Lecturer, King's College London

By the time you get to this section of the guide, you should not be asking which statistics to apply to your data. You should know the answer, which should be defined in your research proposal, driven by your key research question. It is a good idea to enter the data for your study and keep current with the coding as you test the infants or children. By keeping current, not only will you be able to assess whether you are getting positive results but also you may detect problems that you did not anticipate. When computing statistics, first get an overall sense of your data.

You do not want to send an email to your advisor that reads "Dear Professor, there is (or is not) a significant difference—here is the ANOVA." Before you compute the relevant statistics, you should examine such descriptive statistics as the means. Take a careful look at both your highest and lowest scores. Do these scores fall within reasonable parameters? For example, did one child gaze at an object for 20 seconds while another took only 2 seconds with the same object?

Always double-check and then triple-check your data before you even begin thinking about running statistics. Look at your descriptive statistics with your hypothesis in mind. Does everything make sense? Were any variables completely inverted in terms of their expected influence? Always play devil's advocate with your research peers and even with in your deliberations. If you are computing statistics, do your F values correspond with the number of participants in your study manuscript? Does every statistical result make sense? Just because a statistic is generated by a computer, do not assume that it is necessarily correct.

Step back!

What variables are you attempting to assess in your analysis? Does the output of your SPSS/data file make sense? If you are comparing how long infants look at a novel object versus a familiar object and whether there is a significant difference between these two time periods, how many p values would you expect? If you expect three p values, what analysis are they for, and why? If you are assessing whether there is a significant difference between two groups' numbers, you would expect one p value. Step back, question every number you see, and try to comprehend the logic implied by your statistical outputs. Do not send your colleagues random batches of SPSS outputs and Excel files that are not labeled. Rather, date all of your files in the top-right corner, and describe what each analysis means. **A file labeled simply "Output246" can be very dangerous for a variety of reasons.**

 If you happen to have computed statistics for practice or because you were "just curious," be sure to delete these from your computer.

"Do I understand which statistics I should compute—and why?"

"Did I date and clearly label my files/output?"

"Did I compute all relevant descriptive statistics?"

"Did I search out any outliers or inconsistencies?"

"Did I plot a sample graph just to get a feel for the data?"

"Did the inferential statistics I computed fit the patterns suggested by the descriptive statistics and graphs?"

Look for the basic insights implied by your data. If you do compute a significant ANOVA and find, for example, that your children looked significantly longer at the red square than the blue one, specifically how many children followed this tendency? You may end up publishing a research paper based on these data, and any perceived shortcomings could conceivably damage your reputation.

Always be critical. Was anything else going on that might have affected the overall validity of your study results? For instance, you would want to assure in advance that Observer 1 did not test all 5-year-olds and Observer 2 all 10-year-olds. Otherwise, if your data end up indicating an age effect, it might arguably be attributable to differences in the tester. You also should keep the testers and the parents (and participants) uninformed as to your experimental hypotheses so as to minimize bias in their administration of the tests. You should try to assure that parents not influence their children's behavior unduly. One way to do this is by having them wear opaque glasses or simply observe their children through a one-way mirror. You should always strive for generalizability of your results whenever possible. For instance, if your sample is solely children at an elite prep school that costs $65K a year, your results would not likely be generalizable to all children. Similarly, external validity often becomes an issue when testing young infants. At times, some 50% of infants fail to make it through a study for one reason or another (fussiness, excessive movement, experimental error, etc.). In this case, you might want to assess the research literature if possible and explain in your paper that the experienced dropout rate was typical for this type of study (if indeed it was).

O versus 0

Be sure to label and code variables carefully in your files so that there is no ambiguity in understanding them. Be consistent with the terms that you select. Remember that someone may seek to examine the data file that you developed some 20 years from now. I once had a student distinguish infants in two conditions by placing a triangle or a circle next to each infant's name. Not only did the failure to formally define the symbols mean that no one would know what they meant 10 years later (or for *ever*, for that matter), but moreover triangles and circles look all too similar (as opposed to *X*s and an *O*). There was just too much room for potential error. The lesson is to always write and mark clearly and consistently on your coding sheets and logs, as it is important not to leave any room for ambiguity. Also, do not assume that someone will know that 0 means "no" and 1 means "yes" in your data files. Display clear descriptions for any notations used so that anyone will know immediately what a given code means.

What statistic should I compute?

To answer this question, return to your proposal and look up "What is my question?" There are great sources available for those seeking to learn about the bases as well as current trends in statistics. To be on the safe side, you should also consider working closely with and publishing with a professionally trained statistician. Statisticians often bring expertise to bear that developmental scientists lack. They keep up with the latest methods and trends in the field and can help a great deal in deciding what to do about the small sample sizes or missing data points often encountered when researching children.

 Statisticians often make for great collaborators. Involve your statistician in your research project from the start and in your publications if possible. Your statistician is not just a number cruncher or someone to run to when SPSS gives you an output that you do not like. Your statistician likely cares deeply about your research question. Plan a strategy to get him or her involved in your research from the start.

What is the key to working with researchers? What should I remember when working with a statistician?

To address these questions, I asked my collaborator and statistician Dr. Daniel Stahl, Senior Lecturer in Biostatistics at King's College London.

1. Make a plan for how the data will be stored and how data will be analyzed, especially if you have missing data, which is very common for longitudinal studies!
2. Take randomization seriously, and try to do as much blinded as possible.
3. Talk with a statistician *before* you start the study.
4. Don't think that statistics did not advance in the last 50 years!
5. Don't measure everything possible without having a reason for it. You will get too many false positive results.

Any tips on how to plan how many participants will be needed in my study?

Again, from Dr. Stahl:

> Think of what kind of mean score you expect at the beginning (use perhaps pilot data or published data from similar studies), and define the minimum change you would consider as important. Do a simple power analysis for this change (post–pre) or, if you compare two groups, the difference: (post–pre of group 1) – (post–pre of group 2). You can do a simple power analysis based on a t-test (paired for situation 1 and independent for situation 2) using any sample size calculation software such as G*power or Nquery. Estimate how many subjects you expect to drop out, and add this number to your sample size. In general, you should have at least 25–30 subjects per group so that you do not have to worry too much about distributional assumptions.

How do I manage missing data points?

Once more, from Dr. Stahl:

> One way is by using multilevel modeling/mixed modeling. This is now possible to perform in most all software packages including SPSS (mixed model module). Remember to check if the participants who are missing differ in baseline variables and demographics as compared to completers. It will help you to identify if the missing participants have something in common, such as tend to be male or if they have a common social background. It will tell you if you still can generalize your results to the whole population. If a variable predicts missingness, include it in your model as a sensitivity analysis.

Summary (check off your achievements)

- Develop a suitable plan for storing your data. _____
- Reduce the possibility for error by making all your records clear and straightforward. _____
- Always double-check your data entry with fresh eyes. _____
- Know which statistics you will compute before you begin your study. _____
- Measure only what the question posed by your study requires. ____

- Keep up to date on developments in statistics. _____
- Collaborate with a statistician whenever possible. _____
- Label all your files clearly and consistently. _____

EXERCISES

1. Find eight graphs in the news. Present these graphs to your class or your lab. Would you change these graphs—and, if so, in what ways?

_____

_____

_____

_____

_____

_____

_____

_____

2. Find three research papers. Examine all the figures and graphs used. Are the graphs labeled properly? Would you change these—and, if so, in what ways?

_____

_____

_____

_____

_____

_____

_____

_____

3. Take the average of males = 5, 28, and 52 seconds and females = 22, 17, and 42 seconds. Plot a bar graph of mean seconds, with seconds on the *x* axis.

CHAPTER 9
Writing Up Your Research

Before you begin writing up your research, you may want to consider where to submit your paper once it is completed. As you read this chapter, you might also refer to Chapter 10, on selecting a journal and establishing authorship. In the current chapter, I provide several sections of a research paper I coauthored that was published in *PLoS ONE* (June 11, 2008). Here I highlight some of the tips discussed in this guide. Note that the formatting of this research paper follows the specific guidelines of the journal. You should check in advance with the journal where you are submitting your research paper to obtain their formatting requirements. It is also important to remember, as you conduct your research and read published papers, that just because something is published does not mean it is perfect. You might well end up going back to your published work some day and asking, "And why did I write it that way?" Why did I present that graph that way? Just remember that, even if your work is published, there is always room for improvement.

Young Infants' Neural Processing of Objects Is Affected by Eye Gaze Direction and Emotional Expression

Stefanie Hoehl ^

Lisa Wiese ^

&

Tricia Striano *

^ Neurocognition and Development Group, Max Planck Institute for
Human Cognitive and Brain Sciences, Leipzig, Germany
* Hunter College, CUNY, New York City, USA

Correspondence to:
Stefanie Hoehl and Tricia Striano
E-mail: tstriano@hunter.cuny.edu
695 Park Avenue
Hunter College
New York, New York

ABSTRACT

Eye gaze is an important social cue which is used to determine another person's focus of attention and intention to communicate. In combination with a fearful facial expression eye gaze can also signal threat in the environment. **The ability to detect and understand others' social signals is essential in order to avoid danger and enable social evaluation. It has been a matter of debate when infants** are able to use gaze cues and emotional facial expressions in reference to external objects.

Here we demonstrate that by **3 months of age the infant brain differentially responds to objects as a function of how other people are reacting to them**. Using event-related electrical brain potentials (ERPs), we show that an indicator of infants' attention is enhanced by an adult's expression of fear toward an unfamiliar object. The infant brain showed an increased Negative central (Nc) component toward objects that had been previously cued by an adult's eye gaze and frightened facial expression. Our results further suggest that infants' sensitivity cannot be due to a general arousal elicited by a frightened face with eye gaze directed at an object.

The neural attention system of 3-month-old infants is sensitive to an adult's eye gaze direction in combination with a fearful expression. **This early capacity may lay the foundation for the development of more sophisticated social skills such as social referencing, language, and theory of mind.**

NOTE: The first sentence of the abstract is broad and clear. The second sentence becomes more specific. The next sentence highlights why this social signal is so important. The authors highlight a gap in the literature when they state, "It has been a matter of debate." New findings are highlighted. The final sentence highlights the relevance of the research for a variety of disciplines.

Introduction

Social referencing is the ability to search for and to use social signals in order to modulate behavior in new or ambiguous situations [1].

NOTE: Broad and clear general sentence. The introduction of a research paper is written like a funnel with larger topic presented first.

Adults constantly make use of social signals like emotional expressions to guide behavior in ambiguous or dangerous situations [e.g., 2, 3]. Often this is done without conscious control or cognitive effort. For instance, fearful faces which may signal threat automatically capture attention [4–6]. An important neural structure underlying this social threat detection system is the amygdala which is sensitive to fearful expressions and also to eye gaze direction in angry and fearful faces [7, 8]. **However, the developmental trajectory that leads to the efficient detection of relevant social signals in human adults has only been investigated in parts.**

NOTE: Highlighting open question.

For decades research showed that infants show social referencing behavior by the end of the first year [see 1 for a review]. For instance, when faced with an ambiguous and potentially dangerous situation, infants turn to their caregivers and use referential emotional cues to adjust their behavior [9–11]. Importantly, the majority of studies in this field have explored infants' behavioral responses toward an ambiguous or threatening stimulus as a function of an adult's emotional expression and often infants were required to locomote [9–11]. **These measures are highly difficult to apply with younger infants, whose scope of actions is limited. However, it is conceivable that infants' attention system can be affected by referential emotional signals even before infants are able to respond on a behavioral level.**

NOTE: Suggesting gap or open area in the literature.

131

Previous research has demonstrated young infants' remarkable social skills. For example, newborns differentiate between direct and averted eye gaze [12]. By 3 months, infants are able to follow another person's eye gaze [13]. At around the same age, shifts of eye gaze bias infants' attention toward cued targets and facilitate encoding of cued objects [14–16]. Infants are also sensitive to emotional expressions in face and voice from a very early age onwards [17–19]. For instance, the positive slow wave of the infant ERP is sensitive to information conveyed by emotional expressions and eye gaze in 4-month-olds [20]. Another important component in the context of infant face processing is the mid-latency negative central (Nc) component on fronto-central channels. The Nc has consistently been related to attentional orienting to salient stimuli [21, 22], and its amplitude is closely associated with attention as measured by heart rate deceleration [23]. In prior ERP studies, the Nc was sensitive to emotional expressions. An enhanced Nc was found for fearful relative to happy faces [24], angry relative to happy faces [25] and angry relative to happy or neutral prosody [26]. Further, an enhanced Nc was found for angry faces with direct compared to averted eye gaze [27]. Together these results indicate that the Nc response is enhanced by threat-related emotional stimuli.

NOTE: Why is this important?

However, no studies have investigated yet whether young infants' neural system is sensitive to another person's expression of fear toward an object. This involves not only perceiving and discriminating the emotional expression. It also requires that infants link the emotional expression to an unfamiliar object on the basis of eye gaze direction. Possibly, this involves an explicit understanding that the emotional expression is aimed at something in the environment in a referential way. However, rather automatic mechanisms are also conceivable. Based on behavioral studies, the understanding that eye gaze is referential has been attributed to infants by 8 to 12 months of age [28, 29]. Referential understanding of emotions has been demonstrated by 12 months of age [10].

We directly investigated whether young infants' neural responses can be affected by an adult's fearful expression and eye gaze when directed at an unfamiliar object.

NOTE: What's new?

To explore this question we chose the measurement of a well-established neural correlate of infants' attention, namely the Nc component of the ERP.

Three visual ERP experiments with healthy infants were conducted in order to explore young infants' sensitivity to eye gaze and emotional expressions that are directed at external objects. In study 1, 3-month-old infants were exposed to adult faces looking toward unfamiliar objects while posing either a fearful or a neutral expression. Following each face–object stimulus the respective object was presented again without the face (Figure 1a).

NOTE: Clear descriptions.

We chose to test this very young age group because infants use eye gaze cues to guide attention and facilitate learning by that age [14–16].

NOTE: Rationale.

We hypothesized that infants would react with an enhanced Nc component to objects that had been gaze cued by a fearful compared to a neutral face before. If the infant brain is able to link the emotional expression to the object through eye gaze direction, no effect of emotion on Nc amplitude should be found if (1) following each face–object stimulus a novel object is presented (study 2; Figure 2a) and (2) eye gaze of the adult is averted away from the object (study 3; Figure 3a).

Results

ERP responses to objects in study 1 are presented in Figure 1b. Objects that had previously been gaze cued by an adult with a fearful expression elicited a substantially increased Nc component on right fronto-central channels when compared to objects that had been looked at by a neutral face.

NOTE: Figures are well described.

For statistical analyses mean amplitude was considered within a time window of 500–700 ms [milliseconds] after stimulus onset. Mean amplitude was averaged across channels within each region of interest, which were defined as follows: left fronto-central (F3, FC3, and C3), fronto-central (FZ and CZ) and right fronto-central (F4, FC4, and C4). For each of the three studies a repeated measures General Linear Model was applied with emotion (fearful/neutral) and region of interest (left/central/right) as within-subject factors. In study 1, the General Linear Model detected a significant interaction between emotion and region of interest, $F_{(2,13)} = 6.63$, $p = 0.005$. Post hoc two-tailed t-tests revealed that on right channel sites the fearful condition elicited the more negative amplitude peak (mean = –9.58; SD = 2.4) than the neutral condition (mean = –2.74; SD = 2.4), $t_{(14)} = -2.94$, $p = 0.011$. This difference was not significant on left, $t_{(14)} = 0.766$, $p = 0.456$ or central channels, $t_{(14)} = -1.41$, $p = 0.179$. Visual inspection of the data suggested that the ERP may be more negative in the fearful condition even before onset of the Nc. Therefore, a peak to trough analysis was conducted with the positive peak of the so-called Pb component (positive before) between 200 and 400 ms and the negative peak of the Nc between 348 and 700 ms. The interaction between emotion and location was still marginally significant, $F_{(2,13)} = 3.141$, $p = 0.060$. A t-test on right channel sites also revealed a significant effect, $t_{(14)} = -2.735$, $p = 0.016$. The difference between peak of the

Pb and trough of the Nc was greater for the fearful (mean = –25.75, SD = 15.0) than for the neutral condition (mean = –21.09, SD = 13.8).

Applying the same General Linear Model and additional t-tests, no effects of emotion or location on amplitude of the Nc were found in studies 2 and 3 with a statistical threshold of $p < 0.05$ (see Fig. 2b and 3b).

We further applied a General Linear Model with emotion (fearful/neutral) and region of interest (left F3, FC3, C3/ central FZ, CZ/ right F4, FC4, C4) as within-subject factors, and study (1, 2, 3) as a between-subjects factor. This was done in order to test our hypothesis that the factor emotion would have a differential impact on mean amplitude of the Nc in study 1 compared with studies 2 and 3. As expected, a significant interaction between emotion, region of interest and study was found, $F_{(2,42)} = 2.506$, $p = 0.048$.

Discussion

Infants allocated increased attention toward objects that were potentially dangerous, namely objects that had been gaze cued by an adult with a fearful expression.

NOTE: New findings clearly stated.

The lateralization of this effect to the right hemisphere is in accordance with previous findings using a similar paradigm with neutral faces [15] and a right-hemispheric bias for face processing in previous ERP studies investigating the Nc component [30].

However, alternative explanations for these results should be taken into account. First, it is conceivable that a fearful face directing eye gaze toward a simultaneously presented object elicits an unspecific arousal which causes infants to direct attention toward any following stimulus. Therefore, in study 2 infants were presented with novel objects after each face–object dyad. No difference was found between conditions in this study, which suggests that infants did not generalize the emotional expression to any subsequent stimulus.

NOTE: Alternative explanations highlighted.

Second, it may be that a fearful face attracts infants' attention away from the object more than a neutral expression. Therefore, when presented again, objects that had been gaze cued by a fearful face may be more novel and attract more attention compared to objects that had been accompanied by a neutral face. Further, it may be that infants simply associated the fearful face with the simultaneously presented object without regarding the adult's gaze direction. In study 3, eye gaze of the adult was therefore averted away from the object. Again, no difference between fearful and neutral trials was found. This suggests that infants were indeed sensitive to the adult's eye gaze direction, and did not react with enhanced attention toward objects that had previously been presented with a fearful face gazing away from the object. The results of this study also speak against the interpretation that infants in study 1 allocated more attention toward fearfully cued objects because these were less familiar. If the presence of a fearful face prevented efficient encoding of objects in study 1 the same effect should have been observed in study 3, which was not the case.

The current experiments are the first to demonstrate 3-month-old infants' sensitivity to fearful expressions together with referential eye gaze.

NOTE: What's new about these findings.

These findings are intriguing considering that previous studies failed to demonstrate social referencing behavior in infants at 10 months [31, 32]. What can account for this discrepancy? Instead of exploring infants' behavioral reactions to displays of emotion directed at novel objects, we chose to measure infants' attention to gaze cued objects as reflected by the Nc component. We show that infants' attention toward novel objects is substantially increased by an adult's expression of fear toward the object. We suggest that even though young infants' scope of action is limited, they are nonetheless already prepared to utilize adults' social signals in order to guide their attentional resources [see also 33, 34].

However, our results leave open whether infants were really aware of the referential meaning of eye gaze and a fearful expression in our experiment. Potentially, the fearful expression elicited an enhanced arousal which was then associated with the gaze cued object. Even without an explicit understanding of the referential meaning of the communicative signals this would lead to enhanced attention toward fearfully cued objects. In either way, we show that remarkably young infants are able to discriminate an emotional from a neutral expression and associate it with a gaze cued object.

The cortical source of the Nc component has been located in the prefrontal cortex and anterior cingulate [35], which is implicated in conflict monitoring and attention control [36–40]. In patients with panic disorders abnormal activations have been found in response to fearful facial affect in the anterior cingulate and the amygdala [41]. The amygdala is known to play a crucial role in the processing of threat-related stimuli [42, 43], and is sensitive to the direction of eye gaze in faces displaying fearful or angry affect [7]. A fearful face directing eye gaze at a novel stimulus may rapidly elicit activation in subcortical structures which then modulate activation in cortical structures related to attentional processes [4]. Our findings suggest that this mechanism may come on-line very early in human ontogeny. Indeed, it has been argued that a subcortical face processing pathway, involving the amygdala, exists already in early infancy, and that this pathway modulates responses of cortical areas to social stimuli [44]. This subcortical pathway may be involved in enhancing infants' attention to faces and socially relevant stimuli [45].

Our findings suggest that even before infants are able to regulate behavior according to an adult's emotional signals toward objects or persons, infants' attention system can already be affected by social cues that signal threat, i.e., a fearful face with eye gaze directed at an object. Further research is required to determine whether this effect is restricted to threat-related emotional expressions like fear and maybe anger, or whether any emotional expression may elicit a similar effect compared with a neutral face. Future studies should also use behavioral measures of attention which have already been applied successfully with young infants [14]. If similar findings can be obtained using different measures of attention this might help to pinpoint the underlying mechanisms.

It has been argued that the ability to detect eye gaze may have evolved in order to detect threat from potential predators [46]. Eye gaze detection is a very basic mechanism that can be observed very early in human ontogeny and that has evolved early in phylogeny. Even nonmammalian prey species, such as black iguanas and chickens, are sensitive to the direction of eye gaze [see 47 for a review]. Primates systematically follow the gaze direction of conspecifics [48] and follow a human experimenter's gaze even behind a barrier [49, 50]. **From an evolutionary perspective the neural mechanisms examined** in this study are highly adaptive as they may directly contribute to survival in potentially dangerous situations.

NOTE: General relevance and breadth which may be relevant for early development, anthropology, neuroscience and affective sciences.

Materials and Methods

Subjects and experiments. Fifteen typically developing infants (age range from 3;0 months to 4;0 months; study 1: average age 112.5 days, 11 males; study 2: average age 103.5 days, 10 males; study 3: average age 112.5 days, 8 males) were included in the final samples of each of the 3 experiments, respectively, after their parents had given written consent. In all, another 58 infants had to be excluded from the 3 experiments due to fussiness or failing to reach at least 10 artifact-free trials per condition for averaging. This corresponds to the common dropout rate in infant ERP studies [51]. The mean number of trials that were included for every infant per condition was 19.06.

NOTE: Explanation for high dropout rate.

Each trial consisted of a central attractor object (displayed for 500 ms), a fearful or neutral face plus object stimulus (displayed for 1500 ms), a blank screen period with a randomly varying duration (400–600 ms) and an object (displayed for 1000 ms). Every trial was followed by a blank screen period, whose duration varied randomly between 800–1200 ms. Original pictures of neutral and fearful stimulus faces from one male and one female actor were taken from the NimStim Face Stimulus Set (*www.macbrain.org*). The irises were moved from the middle to the left and right corner of the eyes using Adobe Photoshop. Stimulus size was 25 cm × 23 cm.

Infants sat on their mother's lap in a dimly lit, sound-attenuated and electrically shielded cabin at a viewing distance of 90 cm away from a 70-Hz 17-inch stimulus monitor. The experiment consisted of one block with 160 trials (containing 80 neutral and 80 fearful face trials). Stimuli were presented using the software ERTS (BeriSoft Corporation, Germany). The two conditions were presented to the infant in a random order with the constraint that the same condition was not presented three times consecutively and that the number of presentations of each set of stimuli was balanced in every 16 trials. The same faces and objects were presented in each of the experiments and in neutral and fearful trials, respectively. Only trials were included in which the infant had seen both the face–object stimulus and the following object. If the infant became fussy or uninterested in the stimuli, the experimenter gave the infant a short break. The session ended when the infant's attention could no longer be attracted to the screen. EEG was recorded continuously and the behavior of the infants was also video-recorded throughout the session.

NOTE: We can almost see the baby in the testing room. We know where the baby is before we know what he/she looks at.

Electrophysiological recordings. The same methods and statistical analyses were applied for each of the three experiments. EEG was recorded continuously with Ag–AgCl electrodes from 23 scalp locations of the 10–20 system, referenced to the vertex (Cz) which were attached to a cap. Data were amplified via a Twente Medical Systems 32-channel REFA amplifier. Horizontal and vertical electro-oculograms were recorded bipolarly. Sampling rate was set at 250 Hz. EEG data were re-referenced offline to the linked mastoids. A bandpass filter was set from 0.3–20 Hz.

The EEG recordings were segmented into epochs of waveform that comprised a 200 ms baseline and 1000 ms of one static image featuring an object. For the elimination of electrical artifacts caused by eye and body movements, EEG data were rejected offline whenever the standard deviation within a 200 ms gliding window exceeded $80\mu V$ at EOG electrodes or $50\mu V$ at any scalp electrode. Data were also visually edited offline for artifacts and matched with the infant's recorded behavior. Only trials were included in which the infant had looked to the screen and displayed no eye movements.

Acknowledgments

We are grateful to the infants and parents who participated, and to the Universitätsfrauenklinik and the Klinikum St. Georg for support and assistance with recruitment.

References

1. Feinman S, Roberts D, Hsieh K-F, Sawyer D, Swanson D (1992) A critical review of social referencing in infancy. In: Feinman S, editor. *Social referencing and the social construction of reality in infancy.* New York: Plenum Press. pp. 15–54.
2. Latané B, Darley JM (1970) *The unresponsive bystander: Why doesn't he help?* New York: Appleton-Century-Crofts.
3. Prentice DA, Miller DT (1996) Pluralistic ignorance and the perpetuation of social norms by unwitting actors. In: Zanna MP, editor. *Advances in experimental social psychology.* San Diego, CA: Academic Press. Vol. 29, pp. 161–209.
4. Morris JS, Öhman A, Dolan RJ (1999) A subcortical pathway to the right amygdala mediating "unseen" fear. *Proc Natl Acad Sci USA* 96: 1680–1685.
5. Vuilleumier, P (2002) Facial expression and selective attention. *Curr Opin Psychiatry* 15: 291–300.
6. Öhmann, A (2005) The role of the amygdala in human fear: Automatic detection of threat. *Psychoneuroendocrin* 30: 953–958.
7. Adams RB, Gordon HL, Baird AA, Ambady N, Kleck RE (2003) Effects of gaze on amygdala sensitivity to anger and fear faces. *Science* 300: 1536.
8. George N, Driver J, Dolan RJ (2001) Seen gaze-direction modulates fusiform activity and its coupling with other brain areas during face processing. *NeuroImage* 13: 1102–1112.
9. Sorce JF, Emde RN, Campos J, Klinnert MD (1985) Maternal emotional signalling: Its effect on the visual cliff behavior of 1–year-olds. *Dev Psychol* 21: 195–200.
10. Moses LJ, Baldwin DA, Rosicky JG, Tidball G (2001) Evidence for referential understanding in the emotions domain at twelve and eighteen months. *Child Dev* 72: 718–735.
11. Vaish A, Striano T (2004) Is visual reference necessary? Contributions of facial versus vocal cues in 12–month-olds' social referencing behavior. *Dev Sci* 7: 261–269.
12. Farroni T, Csibra G, Simion F, Johnson MH (2002) Eye contact detection in humans from birth. *Proc Natl Acad Sci USA* 99: 9602–9605.
13. D'Entremont B, Hains SMJ, Muir DW (1997) A demonstration of gaze following in 3– to 6–month-olds. *Inf Behav Dev* 20: 569–572.
14. Hood BM, Willen JD, Driver J (1998) Adults' eyes trigger shifts of visual attention in human infants. *Psychol Sci* 9: 131–134.
15. Reid VM, Striano T, Kaufman J, Johnson MH (2004) Eye gaze cueing facilitates neural processing of objects in 4-month-old infants. *NeuroReport* 15: 2553–2556.
16. Reid VM, Striano T (2005) Adult gaze influences infant attention and object processing implications for cognitive neuroscience. *Europ J Neurosci* 21: 1763–1766.
17. Walker-Andrews AS (1997) Infants' perception of expressive behaviors: Differentiation of multimodal information. *Psychol Bull* 121(3): 437–456.
18. de Haan M, Nelson CA (1998) Discrimination and categorization of facial expressions of emotion during infancy. In: Slater AM, editor. *Perceptual development: Visual, auditory, and language perception in infancy.* London: University College London Press. pp. 287–309.
19. Leppänen JM, Nelson CA (2006) The Development and Neural Bases of Recognizing of Facial Emotion. In: Kail R, editor. *Advances in child development and behavior.* London: Elsevier Press. Vol. 34, pp. 207–246.
20. Striano T, Kopp F, Grossmann T, Reid VM (2006) Eye contact influences neural processing of emotional expressions in 4–month-old infants. *Soc Cogn Affect Neurosci* 1(2): 87–95.

21. Courchesne E, Ganz L, Norcia AM (1981) Event-related brain potentials to human faces in infants. *Child Dev* 52: 804–811.
22. Nelson CA (1994) Neural correlates of recognition memory in the first postnatal year of life. In: Dawson G, Fischer K, editors. *Human behavior and the developing brain.* New York: Guilford Press. pp. 269–313.
23. Richards JE (2003) Attention affects the recognition of briefly presented visual stimuli in infants: An ERP study. *Dev Sci* 6: 312–328.
24. Nelson CA, de Haan M (1996) Neural correlates of infants' visual responsiveness to facial expressions of emotion. *Dev Psychobiol* 29(7): 577–595.
25. Grossmann T, Striano T, Friederici A (2007) Developmental changes in infants' processing of happy and angry facial expressions: A Neurobehavioral Study. *Brain Cogn* 64: 30–41.
26. Grossmann T, Striano T, Friederici AD (2005) Infants' electric brain responses to emotional prosody. *NeuroReport* 16(16): 1825–1828.
27. Hoehl S, Striano T (2008) Neural processing of eye gaze and threat-related emotional facial expressions in infancy. *Child Dev* 79(6): 1752–1760.
28. Woodward AL (2003) Infants' developing understanding of the link between looker and object. *Dev Sci* 6(3): 297–311.
29. Csibra G, Volein A (2008) Infants can infer the presence of hidden objects from referential gaze information. *Brit J Dev Psychol* 26(1): 1–11.
30. de Haan M, Johnson MH, Halit H (2003) Development of face-sensitive event-related potentials during infancy: A review. *Int J Psychophysiol* 51: 45–58.
31. Walden TA, Ogan TA (1988) The development of social referencing. *Child Dev* 59: 1230–1240.
32. Mumme DL, Fernald A (2003) The infant as onlooker: Learning from emotional reactions observed in a television scenario. *Child Dev* 74: 221–237.
33. Csibra G, Gergely G (2006) Social learning and social cognition: The case for pedagogy. In: Munakata Y, Johnson MH, editors. *Processes of Change in Brain and Cognitive Development: Attention and performance XXI.* Oxford: Oxford University Press. pp. 249–274.
34. Reid VM, Striano T (2007) The directed attention model of infant social cognition. *Eur J Dev Psychol* 4: 100–110.
35. Reynolds GD, Richards JE (2005) Familiarization, attention, and recognition memory in infancy: An event-related potential and cortical source localization study. *Dev Psychol* 41: 598–615.
36. Casey BJ, Trainor R, Giedd J, Vauss Y, Vaituz CK (1997) The role of the anterior cingulate in automatic and controlled processes: A developmental neuroanatomical study. *Dev Psychobiol* 30: 61–69.
37. Bush G, Luu P, Posner MI (2000) Cognitive and emotional influences in anterior cingulate cortex. *Trends Cogn Sci* 4: 215–222.
38. Duncan J, Owen AM (2000) Common regions of the human frontal lobe recruited by diverse cognitive demands. *Trends Neurosci* 23: 475–483.
39. Botvinick MM, Cohen JD, Carter CS (2004) Conflict monitoring and anterior cingulate cortex: An update. *Trends Cogn Sci* 8: 539–546.
40. Crottaz-Herbette S, Menon V (2006) Where and when the anterior cingulate cortex modulates attentional response: Combined fMRI and ERP evidence. *J Cogn Neurosci* 18: 766–780.
41. Pillay SS, Gruber AS, Rogowska J, Simpson N, Yurgelun-Todd DA (2006) fMRI of fearful facial affect recognition in panic disorder: The cingulate gyrus-amygdala connection. *J Affect Disord* 94: 173–181.

42. Adolphs R (2002) Neural systems for recognizing emotion. *Curr Opin Neurobiol* 12: 169–177.
43. LeDoux J (2003) The emotional brain, fear and the amygdala. *Cell Mol Neurobiol* 23: 727–738.
44. Johnson MH (2005) Sub-cortical face processing. *Nature Rev Neurosci* 6: 766–774.
45. Gliga T, Csibra G (2007) Seeing the face through the eyes: A developmental perspective on face expertise. *Prog Brain Res* 164: 323–339.
46. Haxby JV, Hoffmann EA, Gobbini MI (2002) Human neural systems for face recognition and social communication. *Biol Psychiatry* 51: 59–67.
47. Emery NJ (2000) The eyes have it: Neuroethology, function and evolution of social gaze. *Neurosc Biobehav Rev* 24: 581–604.
48. Tomasello M, Call J, Hare B (1998) Five primate species follow the visual gaze of conspecifics. *Anim Behav* 55, 1063–1069.
49. Tomasello M, Hare B, Agnetta B (1999) Chimpanzees follow gaze direction geometrically. *Anim Behav* 58: 769–777.
50. Bräuer J, Call J, Tomasello M (2005) All great ape species follow gaze to distant locations and around barriers. *J Comp Psychol* 119: 145–154.
51. Leppänen JM, Moulson MC, Vogel-Farley VK, Nelson CA (2007) An ERP study of emotional face processing in the adult and infant brain. *Child Dev* 78: 232–245.

Figure Legends

Figure 1. Stimuli and results for study 1. Example of one trial in the fearful face condition (Figure 1a). A central attractor object preceded each trial to catch infants' attention. Then a fearful or neutral face was presented looking at an object. A blank screen period followed after the face and object stimulus (not depicted, varying duration between 400 and 600 ms). The same object was then presented alone, followed by a blank screen period. Note that the depicted face was not used in the current study. Original faces cannot be published.

ERP responses to objects alone on fronto-central channels (Figure 1b). Note that negative is plotted upwards. Objects that had before been gaze cued by a fearful expression elicited a substantially enhanced Nc component (gray) compared to neutrally cued objects (black).

Figure 2. Stimuli and results for study 2. Example of one trial in the fearful face condition (Figure 2a). Following each face–object stimulus a different object was presented.

ERP responses to objects alone on fronto-central channels (Figure 2b). Note that negative is plotted upwards. No difference was found between Nc amplitude for objects following a fearful compared to a neutral face plus objects dyad.

Figure 3. Stimuli and results for study 3. Example of one trial in the fearful face condition (Figure 3a). Neutral and fearful faces gazed away from the objects that were subsequently presented alone.

ERP responses to objects alone on fronto-central channels (Figure 3b). Note that negative is plotted upwards. No difference was found between Nc amplitude for objects that had been presented with a fearful compared to a neutral face gazing away from the object.

1 a)

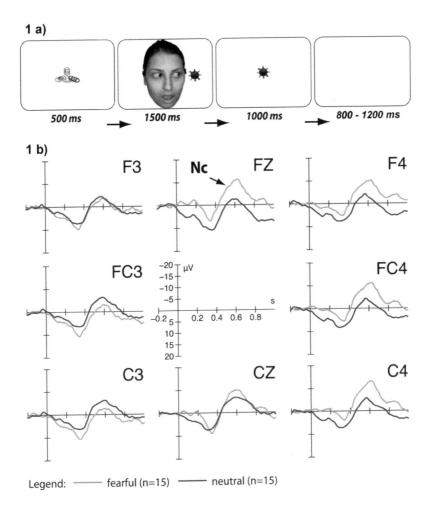

1 b)

Legend: ——— fearful (n=15) ——— neutral (n=15)

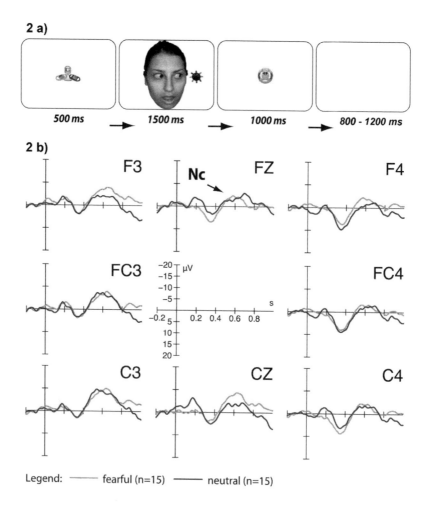

2 a)

500 ms → 1500 ms → 1000 ms → 800 - 1200 ms

2 b)

F3   Nc   FZ   F4

FC3   −20 µV   FC4
−15
−10
−5
s
−0.2 5   0.2 0.4 0.6 0.8
10
15
20

C3   CZ   C4

Legend: —— fearful (n=15) —— neutral (n=15)

3 a)

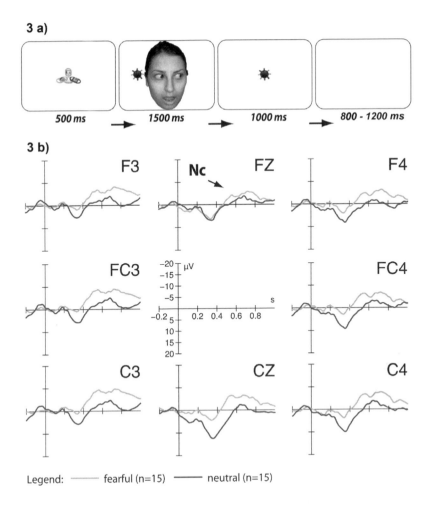

| 500 ms | → | 1500 ms | → | 1000 ms | → | 800 - 1200 ms |

3 b)

Legend: —— fearful (n=15) —— neutral (n=15)

CHECKLIST FOR SUBMITTING YOUR PAPERS
TO YOUR MENTORS AND TO JOURNALS

Overall

_____ I checked the manuscript guidelines for the journal to which I plan to send my paper.

_____ I read two to three papers previously published in this journal, which gave me a sense of the correct formatting and structure to use for my paper.

Editing

_____ I removed all unnecessary words and phrases for my manuscript.

_____ Once I finished writing the paper, I put it away for 1–2 days before rereading it for errors. I also read it again for clarity before sending it to my collaborators/mentor.

_____ I carefully reread the manuscript at least 2 to three times, looking for typos and errors.

_____ I played "devil's advocate," looking for any errors, possible confounds, and logical gaps in my manuscript. I tried to explain any issues still outstanding and back up my views with documentation.

_____ I looked for ways to make transitions within the manuscript smooth and logical.

_____ I confirmed that all my sentences were no longer than two lines (especially for a nonnative audience).

_____ I kept terms in my paper as consistent as possible (e.g., I avoided writing that babies saw an _object_, babies saw the _puppet_, babies saw the _stimulus_, babies saw _it_).

_____ I avoided using acronyms unnecessarily, which helped the paper flow.

_____ I read the paper aloud two to three times, which helped me to hear how it flowed (especially for nonnative readers).

_____ I arranged to have a couple of nonexperts read the paper and confirm that they understood it.

_____ I had at least two native speakers of the language I'm using in the paper confirm its grammatical correctness.

(continued)

_____ I used active verbs and parallel sentence structures wherever possible.

_____ I did not use the words "prove," "believe," or "feel that" in the manuscript.

_____ I had two to three colleagues/peers in the lab review my paper and integrated many of their suggestions into it.

Title Page

_____ I made sure that the title of my paper reflected my original big question and the findings of the study.

_____ I made the title as interesting as possible.

_____ I checked with all the coauthors about their correct affiliations.

_____ I acknowledged funding for the study according to the grant's guidelines (if applicable).

_____ I confirmed that all the sentences in my manuscript were direct and concise.

Introduction

_____ I explicitly addressed: "What's the question, why is the study important, and what's new?"

_____ Any reader could find and circle the "What's the question?" section of my paper.

_____ Any reader could find and circle the "Why is it important?" section of my paper.

_____ Any reader could find and circle the "What is new?" section of my paper.

Discussion

_____ I highlighted my study's limitations within the discussion section of the paper.

References

_____ I checked that the references cited in the manuscript were listed in the reference section.

_____ I checked that all references in the reference section were cited in the manuscript.

_____ I confirmed that the numbers of the references listed corresponded to the ones cited in the text (if applicable).

(continued)

Figures

_____ I included readily understandable figure captions.

_____ I included all my figures and graphs.

_____ I properly labeled the x and y axes on my graph.

_____ I confirmed that the labels for the x and y axes correspond to the figure captions.

_____ I included standard error bars (if required).

_____ I confirmed that my graphs and figures correspond with the data that I presented in the results section of the manuscript.

_____ I made graphs that were clear and easy to read, and the formatting of my graphs was consistent throughout the paper.

_____ I used figures and images to help the reader through the manuscript.

TIP: Use figures to guide the reader. Helpful: "As shown in Figure 1, children gazed significantly longer at the red box as compared to the blue box." Not helpful: "On average, children gazed for 8 seconds at the red box and 59 seconds at the green box (see Figure 1)."

Other

_____ I checked with all my collaborators that they wished to be included as authors before I submitted the manuscript.

_____ I let the authors know that I submitted the manuscript and kept them informed when reviews/comments arrived from the editor.

_____ I asked my coauthors whether they wanted to be sent a copy of the submitted version of the manuscript.

"Dead birds"

This is a wonderful term coined by one of my colleagues and mentors. It refers to the "dead" papers that are proudly delivered to colleagues 6 months or 1, 2, or 3 years after we all know the results and after the paper was "hot" and interesting. It's like a cat that expects the master to be happy when it deposits a "dead bird" at his or her feet. You can avoid bringing your colleagues or mentors "dead birds" by writing your papers up quickly for publication and not losing momentum. Did you just get a new job or just get into graduate school? Are you about to get married? Make it a point to submit your research papers *beforehand*—especially if collaborators or coauthors are involved. Once you get revisions back, follow through immediately. If you delay unduly, someone else may end up taking over your research project!

Losing momentum is a big problem!

I like the suggestion offered by my colleague Professor Dr. Sabina Pauen at Heidelberg University.

> *I find it difficult to handle authorship questions when the students who started running a given study under my supervision already finished their PhD and left the department without having written up a manuscript on "their" study. On the one hand, I would like them to simply write up the study despite the fact that they already finished their appointment. On the other hand, their new occupation often prevents them from doing this, and then I am left with data for a study that I had the idea for and funded, but that someone else claims first authorship on without finding the time to actually write the paper. To handle these situations I decided that every student leaving the department must write up a detailed documentation explaining the organization of the data set that is left behind. He/she is allowed to write a first-author paper until 1 year after leaving our team, but if this does not happen, I claim the data for our group. The student who worked on the study might still be invited to be a coauthor, but only if he/she really contributes to preparing the manuscript.*

I submitted my research paper. Now what?

Once you submit your paper to a journal, the waiting process begins. Depending on the particular journal, the process can take anywhere from 2 days to 4 months. It is rare to have a research paper accepted without any revisions. When your letter comes back from the action editor, try to find about 2 hours to reread your paper along with the reviews.

> *Don't take critical reviews personally. They are likely meant to help you improve your work.*
> —Dr. Stefanie Hoehl, Assistant Professor, Heidelberg University

 Set enough time aside to carefully review comments on your paper.

Depending on how upset or overwhelmed you may feel, you might wait several days before starting this process. With time and experience—especially the more papers that you submit—the process will become very easy.

> *The most important thing I have learned is that, if you want to see your paper published, it is important not to give up after rejection. It is also important not to be hypercritical. It is impossible to make a big discovery every time. And, finally, it is important to not publish everything at any cost. Sometimes it is better to wait, to have more data, and to clarify the question/answer so that understanding of the matter is really enhanced!*
> —Dr. Eugenio Parise, Research Scientist,
> Central European University, Budapest, Hungary

The action editor will usually give you some idea of which suggested revisions are considered critical and which are not. Usually your paper will be routed back to the original reviewers, and so it is important that you address their chief concerns, even if you disagree with and do not make all the recommended changes.

I got the following letter. What should I do?

. . . Thank you for submitting your manuscript to Journal X. Your paper, referenced above, has been reviewed by expert(s) in the field. Based on the comments of these reviewer(s), we regret to inform you that we are unable to accept your manuscript for publication in Journal X. . . .

The comments of the reviewers are included below in order for you to understand the basis for the decision, and we hope that these comments will help. . . .

This is a commonly received letter, unfortunately. One thing to always remember is to celebrate properly when you get *good* news from a journal. The best thing to do in this case, however, is to read the comments carefully, and then try to improve your paper by integrating those that you think are important. Assuming there is no *major* work to be done (i.e., necessitating additional research), submit the paper to a different journal.

 Be sure to forward the news (whether good or bad) to your coauthors.

One of the best ways to learn about research and the review process is to get firsthand experience in reviewing papers. Talk to your mentor about helping him or her review papers. You will learn a great deal in the process. Before you know it, papers will be sent directly to you to review (and you may even come to have so many on your desk that you have to decline some).

When your research paper is ready to go to print, you will receive page proofs from the publisher. Carefully review these page proofs, ensuring that there are no errors (large or small) in the paper before it goes off to print. Often you have only a couple of days to make these corrections. Once your paper is in press, feel free to share the word with the parents who participated in your study as well as colleagues and students.

Summary (check off your achievements)

- Address what the question is, why it is important, and what is new. _____

- Read papers in the journal to which you plan to submit your paper (see the next chapter). _____

- Never lose momentum. _____

- Plan ahead! Don't ultimately present your collaborators with a "dead bird." _____

- Carefully read your paper's reviews. _____

- Get experience in reviewing research papers. _____

- Develop a time management plan to revise your paper. _____

- Don't get discouraged. _____

EXERCISES

1. Write an introduction to a research paper. Be sure to include "What's the question, why is it important, and what is new?"

_____

_____

_____

_____

_____

_____

_____

_____

_____

_____

_____

_____

_____

_____

_____

_____

_____

_____

_____

_____

_____

_____

_____

_____

_____

2. Ask a classmate or lab mate to review your introduction. Make three copies and give one to two classmates and a friend. Can they find and circle (1) what's the question, (2) why is it important, and (3) what is new about your study? Did they agree?

_____

_____

_____

_____

_____

3. Write your authorship agreement and project plan here. Discuss it and agree on it with your coauthors, ideally *before* you begin the project.

_____

_____

_____

_____

_____

_____

_____

_____

_____

_____

_____

_____

_____

_____

_____

_____

_____

CHAPTER 10

Selecting a Journal and Establishing Authorship

What happens when I submit my paper to a research journal?

When a manuscript is submitted to a research journal, it most often arrives via email to the computer of the journal editor(s), who then routes the paper to a team of associate/action editors. The action editors oversee the review process and contact potential reviewers. When a research paper is submitted to a journal, it is generally reviewed by two to four scholars in the field who conduct similar research. These reviewers usually have an established track record of having previously published their own research. When you begin writing and submitting research papers for review, you should keep the peer review process clearly in mind. Papers that you see in research journals have been reviewed and accepted by a group of peers. After an initial round of reviews, a research paper is either accepted for publication, accepted pending minor or major revisions, or rejected altogether by the journal. While a minor revision might involve adding some additional statistics or clarifying certain issues, a major one would likely entail conducting additional research. Even after the research team does a major revision, there is no guarantee that their paper will then be accepted for publication. The review process is normally rigorous, helping to ensure that the journal's published papers and data are of high quality.

I'm ready to submit my manuscript.
Which journal should I select?

There is a bit of a science to selecting a journal. In part, the answer to this question depends on how "strong" your paper is and how soon you hope to get it published. Your theoretical orientation may also come into play when deciding upon a journal. Read several papers to get a feel for the journal, and seek out the counsel of a more senior researcher if you are not certain where to submit your paper. As noted in Chapter 5, research journals have different Eigenfactor scores and impact factors, which are often taken as measures of the importance of a given journal. Journals most often list their impact factor on their website.

Here are a few examples: *Child Development* = 4.718, Eigenfactor score .03; *Developmental Psychology* = 3.214, Eigenfactor score .03; *Developmental Science* = 3.888, Eigenfactor score .02. It is important to note that these scores change a bit over the years.

Fast-track options

Some journals permit prospective authors to pick a fast-track option (you would need to check with the journal of interest). This information is most often provided in the journal's submission guidelines. Fast-track submissions are reviewed by one editor and potentially offer prospective authors a fast turnaround time, such as 14–21 days. This can be a great option if you have a strong paper that you would like to see published quickly, but of course it is also risky. The catch is that the paper is either accepted or rejected—with little or no options for revisions, typically. In most cases, if the manuscript is rejected, it can still be resubmitted through the traditional mechanisms, but in the meantime you will have lost valuable time.

You will also want to consider your preferred journal's scope. Does your paper fit within the stated mission and aims of the selected journal? You will also want to examine closely the editorial board of the journal you pick and other papers published there to get a feel for whether that source is right for your paper. If you are submitting the paper with a more senior researcher, ask his or her advice. Often the advice others can provide is invaluable. Also remember that, just because your paper might appear in a journal with lower impact factor, that does not mean it is not exceptional research. Usually all well-nurtured and loved papers eventually find a home.

Keep in mind that when you submit a paper for review a potential reviewer will receive an email that reads something like this:

Subject: Invitation to review

Jan. 6, 2014

Dear Dr. Roberts:

Happy New Year! How are you? I feel guilty asking you this so soon after the holidays, but I hope you will be able to find the time in your busy schedule to assist us with a review of the manuscript "Infants prefer sweet compared to sour flavors," which has been submitted to Journal X.

I am serving as the Action Editor for this submission and I believe your expertise in such areas as social cognition, infant taste preferences, and infant behavior make you the ideal reviewer for this paper. The abstract for the manuscript appears at the end of this letter.

Please let me know as soon as possible if you are able to accept this invitation. To do this, please either click the appropriate link below to automatically register your reply with our online manuscript submission and review system or email me with your reply.

Agreed: click here.

Declined: click here.

Should you accept my invitation to review this manuscript, you will be notified via email about how to access the paper. You will then have access to the manuscript and reviewer instructions. We would like to receive your review within 5 weeks. Thank you for considering this review request from Journal X.

If you are unable to review this paper at this time, we would greatly appreciate your suggesting the names of others who might be able to provide an informed view and evaluation of this submission.

Warm regards,

How do action editors select reviewers?

Generally, editors have a group of guest editors that they regularly call upon. In addition, you might try recommending possible reviewers in your cover letter. You may also request that particular reviewers *not* be selected, particularly where there might be a possible conflict of interest. You will also want to keep in mind many of the dimensions that reviewers are asked to consider when they review your paper. In addition to writing a review that you will see, reviewers are often presented with a checklist (featuring such options as poor, marginal, adequate, good, excellent) that asks them to rank the paper according to such qualities as:

_____ Relevance of the topic

_____ Breadth of the topic

_____ Theoretical framework

_____ Design

_____ Data analysis

_____ Clarity of the writing

_____ Whether it advances knowledge

Keep these points in mind as you are writing your paper. Even if it is considered relevant and well designed, if it is poorly written then chances are that your paper will need to be revised or else it will be outright rejected. There is a great deal of competition at many journals, so do not doom your chances of publication by submitting a paper containing errors.

In most cases, potential reviewers receive only an abstract of your submitted paper. This is why it is so important to write a clear and interesting abstract. An excellent title and well-written abstract can persuade potential reviewers to actually review your paper. The time required to get your research paper reviewed varies greatly. Sometimes you may hear back from an editor in a matter of days, and at other times the process can take several months. If you have not heard back within about 3 months, check with the editor.

What should I include in my cover letter?

Rather than writing a generic cover letter, try to tell the editor briefly what is really new or novel about your research findings and why they might fit best in his or her journal.

We are submitting our paper "Jump for Joy: Children Who Eat Jellybeans Are More Active," for review in Journal _____. Here we show for the first time that 2- to 3-year-old children jump higher after eating jellybeans. These new findings contribute to our understanding of motor development and add to our knowledge of health, nutrition, and early intervention. We look forward to hearing back from you.

Sincerely,

It is important to publish your results in an efficient manner. Part of the research process involves peer review and sharing your research findings with the public. In many cases, research is funded by government or private sources. It is critical to get such sponsored research out to the public in an efficient and timely manner. Your work is not fully done coincident with your thesis or dissertation being complete—not if it is publishable!

Establishing authorship

Seeing a project through from start to finish is crucially important. Keep in mind that researchers often have students who graduate who did not see their study through to publication. Sometimes students return years later asking why they were not included as an author on a subsequent similar study. Do you want to avoid such problems? If so, write up your study quickly, submit it to a journal, and get it published! Return to the time management section of this book (in Chapter 13) if necessary. **It is also a good idea to establish authorship guidelines and include these in your lab's manual or guidelines.** In my lab, generally the person who sees a project through to completion is treated as the primary author. Sometimes there is an individual who conducts a study (and may have even submitted the first version as first author) but later becomes a coauthor if additional studies are conducted and major revisions are needed that the first author did not have time to complete. Do not go "missing in action." It is essential to stay involved with the project until the paper is in print if you wish to be treated as an author.

Summary (check off your achievements)

- Explore journals to submit your paper to, and read published papers in these journals. _____

- Write a clear and meaningful cover letter that highlights your findings or discoveries. _____

- Pay close attention to the journal's guidelines for formatting. _____

- Keep your coauthors informed. _____

- Give your coauthors enough time to provide comments by asking them how much lead time they need. _____

EXERCISES

1. Write a letter to a journal editor here. Have your lab mate or classmate review the letter.

_____

_____

_____

_____

_____

_____

_____

_____

_____

_____

_____

_____

_____

_____

_____

_____

_____

2. Select and read a journal article. Pretend you are a reviewer for the journal. Write your response to the authors. You might even try this exercise for your own research papers.

_____

_____

_____

_____

_____

_____

_____

_____

_____

_____

_____

_____

_____

_____

_____

_____

_____

_____

_____

3. Find the impact factors for six journals not already cited in this book. List the journal, impact factor, and Eigenfactor score below.

1. _____

_____

2. _____

_____

3. _____

_____

4. _____

_____

5. _____

_____

6. _____

_____

4. Find four journals, and list them here. Do these journals have fast-track submission opportunities? What are the page limits or word-count restrictions for each?

1. _____

_____

2. _____

_____

3. _____

_____

4. _____

_____

CHAPTER 11
Communicating Your Research

There are several ways of sharing your research with the public, which is one of the most meaningful rewards of being a scholar and researcher. In addition to publishing our research in peer-reviewed journals, conducting and attending conferences, symposia, and lectures are some of the ways that scientists share research. Presenting the research as a displayed poster at a conference is a common practice prior to submitting the work for publication. It is an excellent way to share one's research with a wider professional audience. Presenting your research at a conference can often inspire you while you are still writing. Sometimes talking about your work with colleagues whom you do not typically see every day can provide fresh perspectives. Do not take any critical comments personally, but rather ponder them carefully and write them down in your notebook. You may, as a consequence, have a better chance to directly address pertinent criticisms and points while you are still writing your manuscript. Also, you never know when someone you spoke with at the conference will end up being the same person who reviews your manuscript for publication. It is often an instructive experience to present your work to colleagues who may have different theoretical positions. You may also have an opportunity to meet distinguished colleagues from around the world.

Develop your poster the same way that you would develop your manuscript. Stand ready to address: What is the big question that you are seeking to answer? Why is this an important question? And what is new about your findings?

When you are at a conference, you may notice that dozens of people congregate around certain posters and relatively few around others. Why is this so? There can be many reasons, but the design of your poster can be one major factor. Make certain that your poster is not too wordy: the fewer words used, the better. Develop an interesting title for your poster. Add a few photos and some clear graphs without too many lines and bars. People may say, "Run me through your poster." You should be able to do this in 3 minutes. First, take a moment to introduce yourself, and get a sense of the person you are presenting to and speaking with. Then, begin: "**The question** I addressed is 'Do 7-month-olds learn from joint attention cues?'" This **is important because** many social and cognitive skills such as language depend on joint attention. Several studies show that infants learn from joint attention cues at 12 months of age [point to the studies on your poster], but no studies have investigated whether younger infants learn from joint attention. In this study, we tested 7-month-olds [**what's new**]. In a between-subjects design, we tested 30 infants in a No-Joint Attention Condition [point to a picture] or a Joint Attention Condition [point to a picture]. We measured infants' looking time and found that they looked longer at an object they had experienced in a joint attention context [point to graph]. Do you have any questions?" At this point, the person examining your poster will either read the additional information on your poster (such as details on how you coded), or they will ask you questions, or they will simply say "Thank you for that wonderful, concise summary" and go on their way. You may also give your visitors a copy of the poster or have a sign-up sheet available so that you can send them additional information. Whatever you do, you do not want to overwhelm your audience with an initial 10- or 20-minute recitation about your poster. Remember to greet the visitors to your poster enthusiastically and with a smile. Also, try to get a good look at their nametag. It can be awkward when someone is talking about your research in the third person because he or she did not take a moment to make proper introductions and get to know you in advance. Always remember that poster presentations are a great way to get to know more people in your field.

POSTERS AND PRESENTATION CHECKLIST

_____ Is the title clear, and does it reflect the theme of my project?

_____ If I'm in a crowded room full of 200 posters, can someone still see or find my poster?

_____ Can someone read my poster readily from a distance of 5 feet?

_____ Do I accurately and concisely describe the research question?

_____ If I had to leave my poster (try not to do this), could someone understand my presentation without my "walking them through it"?

_____ When visitors approach my poster, do I introduce myself clearly?

_____ Did I remember to ask them if they had questions or comments?

_____ Did I include an abstract with a clear take-home message?

_____ Did I show my poster to all my coauthors several weeks before my presentation and ask for comments? (And integrate the comments?)

_____ Did I ask 10 people to read my poster and ask me questions? Were those questions similar? Could I change something in my poster to make it more clear?

_____ Do I have funding to print a $30-poster and to purchase a poster tube? If not, how will I solve this problem (e.g., print the poster on standard paper or hold a fundraiser)?

_____ Is the font consistent?

Are you going to a conference? Try to reach out to researchers that you would like to meet before the conference in order to set up a time to meet for coffee or lunch. Conferences can be very hectic, and you want to maximize the time you spend making new contacts.

Organize a symposium.

Get public speaking and organizational skills experience by organizing a symposium at a conference. First, clearly identify a theme; then, try to develop something truly creative by thinking outside the box and bringing together researchers who are solving a problem in innovative ways (think "interdisciplinary"). Do you want to get to know a particular researcher in the field? Inviting him or her to your symposium is a great way to do it. Be sure to plan ahead. Do not ask someone to join your symposium only 2 weeks before the final registration date, but rather ask well in advance and be specific about what is needed and all the details relating to the event. If the person declines, do not take it personally. Most likely, he or she is already booked or may not even be attending the conference. He or she will be honored that you asked. Examine previous conference guides for inspiration on how best to proceed.

Here is a sample abstract that my students submitted as part of a symposium titled "Understanding Social Meaning: From Non-verbal Cues to Internal States Language: Perspectives from Typical Development and ASD" (Chair: Dr. Roberta Fadda, presented at the International Conference on Infant Studies).

How Babies Understand Playful Intentions in Natural Contexts

Monitoring others' actions and expressions is an important element of social cognition. Children with autism (Philips et al., 1992) often fail to seek relevant social information when they experience another's ambiguous action. By 7 months of age, infants not only look to others when they encounter an ambiguous action, but they also use others' facial expressions to interpret the action (Striano & Vaish, 2006). Selective looking to faces is an important developmental milestone, and dozens of research studies have documented selective looking among infants in the first year. With an eye toward developing better tools that aid parents in detecting early developmental social cognitive milestones, we developed a study to test selective social monitoring in real-world contexts. To determine how robust infants' social monitoring skills are, and to determine if there are optimal contexts for social monitoring, sixteen 8- to 10-month-old infants' selective looking skills were tested in a standard laboratory context and sixteen 8- to 10-month-old infants' selective looking skills were tested outside of the laboratory in public space in New York City. The results will highlight the role of natural context in developing optimal tools for parents and practitioners to assess developmental milestones in the first year.

Things to keep in mind when giving a talk

Giving a talk can often be intimidating, but practice makes perfect. It is important to speak clearly and to provide mainly critical details. One of the most common errors is trying to present too much in one talk. It is often better to describe one to two studies than to tell your audience about every study you ever conducted. Do not assume your audience members are experts in the field, and ideally try to find out as much about them as possible beforehand. A talk that you would give to parents is very different from one you would give at a lab meeting, or a job talk. At the end of the talk, everyone should know the take-home message.

* Keep it simple—no flying text or power points.
* Use a white background with black text for any overhead projections.
* Use a very large font that can be read across the room (by someone older than his or her 20s).
* Remember that "less is more."
* Keep your sentence structures similar (parallel).
* Use Arial or Helvetica font.
* Use note cards if you are nervous (and even if you are not, it's a fine idea).
* Consider: What's the question? Why is it important? What's new (and by extension, what are you going to do about it?)?
* Present well-timed videos, if any.
* Create clear and legible graphs with legends.
* Remember to smile (draw a picture of a smiley face if you might forget!).

- Look up at the audience (don't stare downward).
- Do not lean on the table or lectern.
- Speak slowly.
- Remember that this is not the time to tell the world everything you ever did! Stick to one or two key points and main studies (you will have a chance to talk again in the future).
- Practice, practice, practice (and then practice again).

Your laboratory should have specific guidelines and formats for presenting talks and posters. There are many online resources that may also be of help. Here are just a few, to get some inspiration:

- *www.garrreynolds.com/preso-tips/design*
- *noteandpoint.com/documents/pdf/wwlg.pdf*
- *www.powerpointninja.com/design-tips/powerpoint-design-principle-3-contrast-2*
- *www.sc.edu/cte/guide/powerpoint*
- *www.presentationzen.com/presentationzen/2007/08/i-spent-the-wee.html*

I've been asked to write a public summary. What should I include?

Often, when you receive a grant, you will be asked to write a summary for the public. Just as when you write a paper or proposal, remember to begin with a general overview and then provide more specific details. In many cases, the agency that is requesting a public summary will send you specific guidelines. Here is a published public summary that my laboratory once used; you may want to use it as a model. Just as when you are writing a research paper, the summary begins with a general broad problem. The summary then becomes more specific. Be sure to address how the study solves a relevant problem.

The following is an example of a 2008 public summary for the National Science Foundation.

A quick glance at someone's face can provide essential information. It gives us clues about their internal mental states and future behavior. Humans are surrounded by more information than they can possibly attend to and process. Sensitivity to relevant social cues helps us to determine the importance of information in the world. Among the many types of social cues used in this process, eye gaze is a social cue to which humans often pay close attention. Although our basic understanding of eye gaze perception and processing has increased in past years, the early development and underlying mechanisms of eye gaze processing remain largely unknown. The goals of this project are to assess how social cues influence infants' attention, object processing, and underlying neural processes. With support from the National Science Foundation, Dr. Tricia Striano and colleagues at Hunter College, The City University of New York, will address these questions, using measures of infant brain activity. A series of studies will be conducted in which 3- to 9-month-old infants view computer displays of an adult who is looking away at objects or away at an external location. Changes in electrophysiological brain responses will tell us how neural processing and learning about faces and objects is influenced by eye gaze directionality in early infancy.

The research will broaden our knowledge of infant social-cognitive and brain processing. The research will increase our understanding of infant learning and provide information about how infant learning can be facilitated by social cues. These advancements will be important to provide typically developing infants with optimal learning environments, and eventually to be able to detect atypical social development, as in autism spectrum disorders much earlier. Early identification of autism spectrum disorders is critical for the implementation of more effective early interventions. By involving young scientists in research, the project will also enhance the infrastructure for developmental social neuroscience and autism research at Hunter College, a minority-serving institution. Funding from this application will also allow us to educate the public about early infancy research through dissemination of findings through our website, *www.howbabieslearn.com*; various public talks and events; and a newly developing journal supported in part by Hunter College (*Infancy Research: A Journal for Students, Parents, and Educators*). During the first postnatal year of life, infants acquire skills and knowledge that are foundational for later language acquisition, social-communicative behavior, and cognitive development. The funded project will obtain new information on typical early social development and its impact on infant learning to understand the implications of developmental disorders and environments that may deprive infants of critical learning experiences.

I have received a press inquiry and the following email. What should I do?

I am a science journalist for _____, and I´m preparing an article on early child development. I would be especially interested in your opinions about new publications. Since I have to write my article soon, it would be nice if you told me whether an interview early next week would be possible. Thank you so much for your help!

Working with the media can be a great way to promote your research. However, check when and where the article is being published. It is also a good idea to ask to see your transcribed comments beforehand, given that these might possibly be taken out of context. If the media would like to film your lab, be sure that it is worth the time. Do you really want to stop your research for 10 hours for a camera crew? It may well be worth it, but it depends; so, be sure to get the facts. Be sure to see how it all fits into your time management plan.

What are some other ways to communicate your research?

Developing a laboratory newsletter or blog can also be a great way to communicate your research findings and also to attract increased interest to your laboratory. Articles written by various laboratory members are one way to communicate lab findings and news. If you are part of a small laboratory, try to partner up with another laboratory to enhance mutual efforts at communicating with the local community and beyond.

I'm planning a study with colleagues abroad. What problems should I anticipate? What advice can you offer?

To help to address this question, I turned to one of my colleagues, Christine Michel, a graduate student at Heidelberg University. She was amazing when conducting a research study across continents!

A basic problem refers to language problems, which can certainly lead to misunderstanding. It is helpful to check often [whether] agreements were understood in the same way on both sides. Writing down these agreements can also help.

Another very important topic refers to the problem of data storage and sharing data between both parties. Data should be stored in a way that both sides can have access to it (e.g., in the cloud). Data should always be updated so that both sides are on the same page and in synch.

Both sides should inform each other about cultural and IRB specifics in their country. Problems can be avoided if the other side knows about the issues and demands [that] the partner has to grapple with! Communication is the key.

In terms of communication, it is also very helpful to know with whom you are corresponding . . . and how the hierarchy is structured. Skype or online video chat can be a great way to stay in contact!

But, if possible, get to know your collaborators in person. A visit to get in contact with the other side—especially when working abroad—facilitates the communication and working process!

 The more conflict you can avoid and/or handle efficiently, the more time you can spend on your research. Always be polite in emails; try to use a nice greeting, and write in a professional way even if you are upset. "Dear," "Please," "Thank you . . ." (good words to use!).

Dear . . . ,

Thank you for letting me know that . . .

I would like to propose the following solutions:

1.
2.
3.

Again, thank you very much for reaching out to me. Do the suggestions provided above solve the problem? If not, please feel free to get back to me with an alternative arrangement.

Summary (check off your achievements)

- Communicate research with the public, and keep the following in mind: What is the question? Why is it important? What is new about the findings? _____

- Organize a symposium at selected conferences. _____

- Always have a 3-minute summary of your research ready. _____

- Always have a 20-minute summary of your research ready. _____

- Develop a newsletter. _____

- Communicate through the social media. _____
- Keep your participants up to date on upcoming talks and new publications. _____

EXERCISES

1. Select a research paper. Write a public summary of it.

_____

_____

_____

_____

_____

_____

_____

_____

_____

2. Select four research papers. Develop a newsletter or blog based on these articles.

_____

_____

_____

_____

_____

_____

_____

_____

_____

3. Find three to four research summaries in the news or media. Find and read the corresponding original articles. Is the summary consistent with the research findings? In what ways and in what ways not? If not, rewrite the summary(ies) here.

_____

_____

_____

_____

_____

_____

_____

_____

_____

Index

About the Author

Tricia Striano, PhD, is Professor of Psychology at Hunter College of The City University of New York. Her research on infant and child social and cognitive development has been recognized with the Sofja Kovalevskaja Award from the Alexander von Humboldt Foundation and has been supported with grants from the German Research Foundation and the National Science Foundation. Formerly, she served as Director of the Independent Research Group on Cultural Ontogeny at the Max Planck Institute for Evolutionary Anthropology and Director of the Independent Research Group on Neurocognition and Development at the Max Planck Institute for Human Cognitive and Brain Sciences and the Center for Advanced Studies at the University of Leipzig, Germany. The author of over 100 research papers and edited volumes on social cognition, Dr. Striano serves on the editorial board of *Infant Behavior and Development*. Her website is *TriciaStriano.com*.